GUIDE
TO
YOGA

GUIDE
TO
YOGA

Dilys Hartland & Vicky McDonald

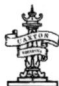

CAXTON REFERENCE

© 2001 Caxton Editions

This edition published 2001 by Caxton Publishing Group Ltd,
20 Bloomsbury Street, London, WC1B 3QA.

Design and compilation by The Partnership Publishing Solutions Ltd,
Glasgow, G77 5UN

Printed and bound in India

Contents

What is Yoga not?   9

Chapter 1 What is Yoga?   11

Chapter 2 Before you start   39
   Why do people learn yoga?   41
   Health Benefits   43

**Chapter 3 An introduction to some basic
            yoga positions**   87

Chapter 4 Yoga and Health Benefits   163
   What is yoga therapy?   165
   Will yoga therapy work for you? 171
   Lack of sleep   174
   Yoga as a benefit for children   186
   Asanas for helping PMS or PMT   188

Pain release through yoga   197

Yoga for MS   205

The use of yoga for facial exercise   210

Chapter 5   Moving on   **215**

Combining asanas   215

Your inner health   217

Lifestyle   219

Meditation   221

Affirmations   224

Visualisation   225

Conclusion   **229**

Useful Addresses   **231**

At the still point
Of the turning world...

Teach us to care and not to care
Teach us to sit still.

T.S. Eliot

What is Yoga not?

This is the best place to start, because this is the easiest question to answer. Yoga is not a painful stretching of the limbs, although efforts are obviously needed to achieve yoga (like everything else).Its goal is not to make us rubber-men and women. It never imposes or forces ideas on anybody or any organisations, rather, Yoga encourages self-investigation, and to see what it can bring us and others, by Ourselves. It is never self-torture. Its goal is not at all to achieve psychic powers, and it will never encourage selfishness or separative attitudes. Most importantly, it is not to be practised only by reading a book.

CHAPTER 1
What is Yoga?

Amongst the subjects covered in this text are ethical living, selfless action, stability of mind, religious duty and lack of desires. It also covers meditation and the nature of the universe and creation. The Yoga Sutras of Patanjali, also known as the Yoga of Eight Limbs, is a philosophical compilation bringing together the complete knowledge about yoga. It is estimated to date from between 200 and 800 BC but it has been considered to be earlier than that by traditional sources.

Yoga is a dynamic system of physical exercise and an extremely valuable philosophy to apply to everyday life. The ultimate goal of yoga philosophy is complete detachment from reality, as we understand it, and complete self knowledge or Samadhi. Only by separating the 'self' part from our environment can we fully come to terms with our individual personality and start putting the mind and emotions in order. This lack of self knowledge is thought to be the fundamental cause of many emotional and nervous problems. Yoga enables us to live our lives at a higher and more fulfilling level.

Most exercise programmes depend mainly on working on the body ignoring the fact that the body and mind have a great effect on each other. Yoga is one of the concepts that could today be described as holistic or in other words affecting the body, mind and spirit i.e. the 'whole' person. The aim of the Yoga teacher is to help pupils to take control of their lives by learning to control the body, breath and mind. The secret is to find a balance in life. It has been said that yoga is not for one who eats too much or too little, not for one who sleeps too much or too little the idea is to achieve moderation in all aspects of ones life. It is often said that you teach what you most need to learn and with this in mind you will find that as well as learning, you will be teaching others your new findings through your personal practice of yoga. We are all individuals and you will find that you will ultimately decide what is right or wrong for you and from this you will learn the best ways of helping yourself overcome certain difficulties and disabilities by adapting Yoga postures accordingly. Yoga is a vast subject which you will go on studying and learning for the rest of your life. The more you can read and explore about Yoga the more interesting it will become. The aim of this book is to give you a firm foundation from which to go on building and developing your skills.

Far too often yoga is practised purely as a physical exercise or to improve ones concentration or ease tension. Whilst it may well be useful for all these purposes, to be successful in yoga the ultimate goal of self realisation must always be the main aim as by working towards this aim we shall be assured of improved concentration, lack of tension etc. However if we are only interested in the side benefits of yoga it is unlikely we shall ever achieve what we set out to do.

The Paths of Yoga, which will be discussed and explained fully later in this chapter, are:

- JNANA YOGA – union by knowledge
- BHAKTI YOGA – union by love
- KARMA YOGA – union by service
- MANTRA YOGA – union by speech meaning recitation of sacred syllables or mantras.
- RAJA YOGA – union by mental control meaning mastery of the mind and senses
- HATHA YOGA – union by bodily control including asanas, kriyas (cleansing processes with water and cloths, pranyamas (these maintain and channel the flow of energy), bandhas (closing actions which prevent energy loss)

No matter which path is followed there are eight essential practices or limbs:

1 YAMA – abstention from evil
- non-stealing
- truthfulness
- non-destruction
- moderation in eating and physical pleasures
- non-desire for possessions of others

2 NIYAMA – observances
- contentment
- study
- cleanliness of mind and body
- strength of character
- self surrender to the Lord

3 ASANA – postures

4 PRANAYAMA – breath control

5 DHARANA – concentration of mind on a particular point or object

6 DHYANA – meditation

7 PRATYAHARA – sense withdrawal from external world into the interior self

8 SAMADHI – self realisation

Today, yoga tends to be known as a technique of keeping fit and supple and for toning your muscles. It is also known to be a spiritual, peace-generating practice. The very ancient custom of yoga is at least several thousand years old and the very first references to it have been found and studied in the

Vedas , which are the sacred writings of Hinduism between the years of 3000 BC and 1200 BC. Its place of origin was in India, in fact in what is now known as Pakistan. However, there are some sources that describe the art as being introduced by ancient Tibetan monks as a form of meditation and relaxation. The art of yoga as we know it today thus pre-dates Christianity by thousands and thousands of years, and in the East, people were practising their form of yoga when Western civilisations barely existed at all.

In India, Yoga is seen as one of the six branches of classical philosophy, and is encapsulated in a set of aphorisms collated and organised by Patanjali in the Yoga Sutras. The word Yoga derives from the Sanskrit, meaning to bind, to join, to yoke as well as union or communion.

There are 8 stages (or limbs) of yoga which must be followed in order to reach Samadhi, the last stage, where the spirit is liberated and joins the Universal Spirit.

Yoga is a dynamic system of physical exercise and a valuable philosophy to apply to everyday life. The ultimate goal of yoga philosophy is complete detachment from reality, as we understand it, and complete self knowledge or Samadhi. Only by separating yourself from the environment can you come to terms with your individual personality and start putting the mind and emotions in complete order. This lack of self knowledge is thought to be the fundamental cause of many emotional and nervous problems. Yoga aims to deal with that and put it to right.

The word 'yoga' comes from the ancient Sanskrit language and means union. There are various yoga systems but the goal is always the same, which as I have said, is perfect self knowledge. The most popular form of yoga practised in this country is Hatha yoga which is concerned with body control and consists of a series of exercises or asanas. The word Hatha is made up of HA meaning sun and THA meaning moon. Through the practice of Hatha, the body is enlivened by many positive and negative currents and when these are in complete equilibrium, the theory is that we enjoy perfect health. Although Hatha yoga is essentially concerned with the control of the body, it has a much wider effect as in a fit body all systems will function efficiently, which will in turn help to calm the mind. About 2500 years ago Buddha stated 'you are what you think' and Patanjali, considered to be the father of traditional yoga, defined yoga as being the controller of the activities of the mind. Most exercise programmes depend mainly on working on the body, but ignore the very major fact that the body and mind have a great and distinct effect on each other. Yoga is one of the concepts that could today be described as holistic or, in other words, affecting the body, mind and spirit i.e. the 'whole' person. Yoga helps people to take control of their lives by learning to control the body, breath and mind. The secret is to find a settling balance in life. It has been said that yoga is not for one who eats too much or too little, not for one who sleeps too much or too little. The overall idea is to achieve moderation in all aspects of ones life. Many types of exercise require expensive apparatus and are dependent on other people whereas Yoga only needs a certain amount of time and ones desire to practice.

Far too often yoga is practised purely as a physical exercise or to improve ones concentration or ease tension. Whilst it may well be useful for all these purposes, to be successful in yoga the ultimate goal of self realisation must always be the main aim as by working towards this aim we shall be assured of improved concentration, lack of tension etc. However if we are only interested in the side benefits of yoga it is unlikely we shall ever achieve what we set out to do.

The tradition of yoga was originally handed down orally as teachings with a guru - or a teacher - passing on his great and respected knowledge to his pupils, and this master to pupil tradition continued for many generations. When Prince Gautama Siddhartha left his life of great luxury and privilege at an Indian court to seek spiritual enlightenment, sometime around 530 BC, he sat in meditation under a banyan tree looking for inner freedom. He achieved enlightenment through the practice of the art of yoga, and went on to found one of the world's great religions – that of Buddhism. The first written account of yoga, however, dates from the 2nd century BC, when the Indian sage, known as Patanjali, described the 'system' of yoga in a long and detailed document called the Yoga Sutras. Patanjali described what are known as The Eight Limbs of Yoga, which are practices which a man should follow in order to become a yogi and achieve great wisdom. A yogi is one who practices yoga in its fullest and most developed sense.

The Eight Limbs, or steps, described by Patanjali are:

1 Yama

This stage is known to be the adherence to all of the principles such as non-violence, chastity or fidelity and truth-telling, and neither stealing nor coveting, that is lusting after the acquisition of material possessions. It is the bringing together of the universal moral commandments, similar to western moralities – non-violence, truthfulness, non-stealing and non-coveting.

2 Niyama

This is the second stage and describes the disciplines or 'observances' which are necessary to be a wise person. These factors are purity, contentment, austerity, study and devotion to the Universal Being – in other words, God in whatever form you perceive God to be. In other words, it is the rules of conduct applicable to the self, such as purity, contentment, ardour, self-study and dedication.

3 Asanas

This Limb is the study of bodily postures. Literally, an asana is 'a steady pose'. These positions are, of course, what we in the Western world typically tend to think of as being the art of yoga. In fact, as you see, they are only one branch of a much wider, philosophy which encompasses a much greater area and artform.

There are said to be many thousands of asanas. Again, modern Western yoga uses comparatively few of these positions and uses them in a basic form. Many of the asanas have different grades of difficulty, with a variation of postures that can be added to the basic core pose, according to the flexibility and the experience of the practitioner.

4 Pranayama

This branch concentrates on the study of breath control, or purposeful and regulated breathing. It is the rhythmic control of breathing, and is generally only taught in the West to more accomplished students.

5 Pratyahara

This step is the withdrawal of the senses.

6 Dharana

This is the concentration branch of the individual.

7 Dhyana

This branch studies and deals with the practice of meditation in conjunction with the positions of yoga.

8 Samadhi

This has been variously described as illumination, self-awareness or a heightened state of consciousness.

In general, the West has mainly accepted the practice of asana and pranayama, enabling the body to be healthy and free from stress and illness. Thus, to a certain extent, yoga in the West is closely related to the idea of living a good and healthy life. It stands in contrast to the acquisitiveness and high pace of modern life and can provide the student with a framework for making sense of their life. Modern western life has brought tremendous benefits but also its own perils. The elimination of the drudgery in our lives has left us with an immobile, sedentary lifestyle, where the intellect holds sway over the body in the pursuit of happiness. But the lack of natural exercise in our lives has left many people with chronic health and stress problems, especially as they get older. Yoga enables the student to find relief from these physical ailments and to strengthen the body and make it more supple.

Regular asana and pranayama practice will bring serenity and calmness to the student, enabling the internal organs to become strong and to work efficiently. By so doing the student can overcome many symptoms of stress, such as headaches, stiff necks, lower backache, insomnia and digestive disorders. Yoga practice helps to improve concentration and self-discipline, and to harness one's energy – by so doing, it brings vitality in your everyday activities.

From the psychological viewpoint, yoga sharpens

the intellect and aids concentration. It steadies the emotions and encourages a caring concern for others. Above all, it gives hope. The practice of breathing techniques calms the mind. Its philosophy sets life in perspective. In the realm of the spiritual, yoga brings awareness and the ability to be still. Through meditation, inner peace is experienced. Thus yoga is a practical philosophy involving every aspect of a person's being. It teaches the evolution of the individual by the development of self-discipline and self-awareness. Anyone, irrespective of age, health, circumstance of life and religion, can practise yoga.

It was not expected that a man – and it always was men who practised yoga – would concentrate his yoga on one limb and then go on to work on another. All eight steps represent the paths which a man must follow simultaneously in order to achieve the wisdom they desire – they are the foundations of a more complete way of life. All eight practices make up the tradition of yoga but, as we have seen, our Western view of it has narrowed it down to just two paths: those of bodily posture (the individual yoga postures are called asanas) and the breath control (pranayama) that accompanies it. Occasionally, meditation becomes involved, but meditation and yoga are often seen as being two separate arts, rather than two practices that can be done together to enhance their results.

Yoga is neither a religion nor a political belief. You could happily and beneficially practice yoga from today for the rest of your life without subscribing to any set of rules or regulations. You don't have to join anything (except perhaps a class) or give money to any particular cause. Because of its ancient origins it has strong associations with various cultures and faiths (predominantly Hinduism), but if you define any causes with which it has a connection these are the causes of non-violence, of individual fulfilment and of universal peace and harmony.

Sanskrit is the ancient language of yoga and, as previously mentioned, the word 'yoga' itself means 'union'. This signifies the union between mind and body, and between the conscious mind and those unconscious levels that lie beneath it.

Within the entire yoga tradition, there are various ways of practising the Eight Limbs that have developed over many, many centuries. In trying to understand this, it is helpful to think of all the branches of a tree, or the spokes of a wheel or the rays of the sun – they all extend from the same source and are inseparable from that core, but they each still have an individual identity.

Some of these branches are:

Mantra yoga

A mantra is a word, sound or phrase which is repeated over and over and over again until it becomes internalised. The person saying the mantra and the mantra become one. The use of a mantra leads to focus, awareness, heightened consciousness and peace. Most forms of meditation make use of a mantra to still the mind and focus the meditator. This is certainly true of the best-known (but by no means only) form of meditation, the transcendental meditation taught by the Maharishi Mahesh Yogi.

Some yoga classes begin and end with the repetition of the word 'Om', which can be used as a mantra. This is discussed more fully later on.

Bhakti yoga

This is described as the 'devotional' path, and in essence means reflecting on the divine, channelling the emotions into acts of worship. This can take many forms. For instance, one who studies art or music can be said to be reflecting on the divine, since things of beauty and creativity are the works of God (I'm using the word God in the broadest possible sense, of a universal life force or spirit).

Karma yoga

This is the yoga of action. Many people are now

familiar with the law of karma, which is the same as cause and effect: you shall reap what you sow, in Biblical terms. So those who go down the path of karma yoga engage actively with the world, immersing themselves in the service of others, doing good deeds and acting for the benefit of humanity, so that good may return to them.

Jnana yoga

This is a cerebral, intellectual form of yoga (its name comes from the Sanskrit verb 'to know'), whose followers tend to look within themselves; they are thinkers not doers, analysing rather than feeling.

Raja yoga

Raja yoga is often placed under the same umbrella as hatha yoga. Whereas the path of hatha yoga is through physical control and bodily postures, raja yoga (the word raja means 'royal', in the sense of commanding or authoritative) seeks mastery over the mind and the mental processes.

Hatha yoga

If all of the above seems a bit complicated and not really relevant to your desire to acquire flexible joints and a stronger back, it's because I would like to paint a picture of yoga as something broader and deeper than just another form of physical exercise. While it is that, it's important to see it as one part or expression of a whole philosophy, a complete way of life that reaches back thousands of years to ancient races and civilisations, that spans continents as well as centuries, and has driven and influenced the daily lives of millions in all its diverse forms.

Hatha is derived from two Sanskrit words, 'ha' symbolising the sun, and 'tha' symbolising the moon. The sun and moon are seen as representing the opposites in nature: male and female, hot and cold, light and dark. In life, opposites need to be balanced, the tension between them being kept equal, and balance in all its meanings is at the heart of yoga.

It is sometimes hard for those brought up in Western traditions where mind and body are quite separate entities – with an underlying feeling of 'and never the twain shall meet' – to comprehend their essential unity, a belief that is integral to the practice of yoga. Proper care of the body is essential, as the body houses the soul and carries out the 'work' of the spirit. It is therefore completely contrary to the practice of yoga to mis-use or abuse the body in any way – your own, or other people's – whether with drugs, or cigarettes, or alcohol, or simply by neglecting to eat healthful foods and take appropriate amounts of sleep and exercise.

As indicated above, the two threads of hatha yoga are the postures (asanas) and correct breathing (pranayama). Prana is the Sanskrit word for what is elsewhere described as the life force, or chi in Chinese traditions. In yoga, therefore, breathing is not just maintaining life by respiration, but taking in the life force and circulating it round the body in the most efficient manner. Perhaps because many of us lead sedentary lives, slouched over desks all day long and perhaps hunched in chairs or on sofas most of the evening, we have lost the art of deep nasal breathing. Shallow breathing involves only the wind-pipe and the lungs; true breathing has to draw oxygen into the diaphragm and the abdomen, so that the lungs and chest expand and contract fully. Deep breathing is instantly calming; after all, we commonly say 'take a deep breath and count to ten' as a means of soothing someone who is upset or angry.

In order to breathe properly, you must have the correct posture, and vice versa; correct posture cannot be achieved without deep breathing. This means holding the head erect, with the crown of the head pointing at the ceiling or the sky, the chin level, shoulders back and relaxed so that the chest is open, spine straight so that stomach and diaphragm are not cramped or restricted.

You'll notice that many of the yoga asanas have the names of animals: the Cat, the Dog, the Fish. This is no accident. In yoga there is reverence for life but also a sense that humans are only one among many life forms, and by no means superior. On the contrary, animals (and fish) live in harmony with their bodies; in their fluidity and grace of movement, they fully express themselves through their outward forms. Other asanas take the names of practical everyday objects – the Plough, the Bridge – that are tools or amenities for making life simply better.

There are four main paths of Yoga – **Karma Yoga, Bhakti Yoga, Jnana Yoga** and **Raja Yoga**. Each is suited to a different temperament or approach to life. All the paths lead ultimately to the same destination – to union with Brahman or God – and the lessons of each of them need to be integrated if true wisdom is to be attained.

Karma Yoga

The Yoga of Action

It is the path chosen primarily by those of an outgoing nature. It purifies the heart by teaching you to act selflessly, without thought of gain or reward. By detaching yourself from the fruits of your actions and offering them up to God, you learn to sublimate the ego. To achieve this, it is helpful to keep your mind focused by repeating a mantra while engaged in any activity.

Bhakti Yoga

The Path of Devotion or Divine Love

This path appeals particularly to those of an emotional nature. The Bhakti Yogi is motivated chiefly by the power of love and sees God as the embodiment of love. Through prayer, worship and ritual he surrenders himself to God, channelling and transmuting his emotions into unconditional love or devotion. Chanting or singing the praises of God form a substantial part of Bhakti Yoga.

Jnana Yoga

The Yoga of Knowledge or Wisdom

This is the most difficult path, requiring tremendous strength of will and intellect. Taking the philosophy of Vedanta the Jnana Yogi uses his mind to inquire into its own nature. We perceive the space inside and outside a glass as different, just as we see ourselves as separate from God. Jnana Yoga leads the devotee to experience his unity with God directly by breaking the glass, dissolving the veils of ignorance. Before practising Jnana Yoga, the aspirant needs to have integrated the lessons of the other yogic paths – for without selflessness and love of God, strength of body and mind, the search for self-realisation can become mere idle speculation.

Raja Yoga

The Science of Physical and Mental Control

Often called the 'royal road' it offers a comprehensive method for controlling the waves of thought by turning our mental and physical energy into spiritual

energy. Raja Yoga is also called Ahtanga Yoga referring
to the eight limbs leading to absolute mental control.
The chief practice of Raja Yoga is meditation. It also
includes all other methods which helps one to control
body, energy, senses and mind. The Hatha-Yogi uses
Asanas, Pranayama, Relaxation and other practices
such as Yamas, Niyamas, Mudras, Bandhas etc.. to
gain control of the physical body and the subtle life
force called Prana. When body and energy are under
control meditation comes naturally.

Different paths of yoga in more detail

Yoga comes from connecting to God, just as the word religion means in western context. There are many schools, which are sometimes referred to as sampradajas which all have different forms of yoga. The aim of all teachings is to guide an embodied spirit in a (non)-personal relationship to God. The theory is that there is no more supreme a being as that which lives within your own heart.

The native yoga paths are a part of the religious practice that we refer to today as Hinduism, but the real importance of vedic culture seems to be that it has enabled native yoga paths to stay in the Indian sub-continent. They have remained unchanged there longer than they have in other locations. It seems as if these philosophies were in fact known all over the world.

No form of yoga is better than the other. There are as many different paths as there are individuals existing. The most common of all forms of yoga is that of reconnecting, the religious or even yoga with God.

Karma Yoga (Bhikshu)

Karma Yoga achieves a union with God through right action and through service (Bhakti Yoga). Karma Yoga can also be summed up in a statement which was made by Sri Bhagavan Krishna in the Bhagavad Gita:

"In worshipping Him with proper actions, a man attains realisation". One key to Karma Yoga is the performance of right action and service for its own sake, without consideration of the immediate or apparent results.

Hatha Yoga

Hatha yoga concerned with the physical and energetic purification and training. Its goal is to bring the physical body into a more than perfect state of health, so that the soul has a fitting vehicle of expression to work through and evolve from. Hatha yoga embraces many practices, including physical postures and breathing exercises (known as pranayama) which also act upon the physical nervous system and ethereal body, which is considered a development of the aspects of the physical body, and brings all the vital energies of the physical and ethereal bodies under conscious control.

Jnana Yoga

Jnana yoga is the yoga of the philosopher and thinker who wants to go beyond the visible, material reality of his life and world. The Jana Yogi finds God through knowledge and understanding. Jnana Yoga is summed up in the Upanishads by the following statement: "In the method of reintegration through knowledge, the mind is ever bound to the ultimate end of existence which is liberation This method leads to all attainments and is ever auspicious."

Kundalini Yoga

Kundalini Maha yoga. is an ancient universal science which has been perfected over thousands of years. Anandi Ma is an advanced disciple of Dhyanyogi yoga and one of few people who can perform Skaktipat. Through Shaktipat the disciple can excel quickly in their spiritual journey towards Self Realisation and enlightenment.

Agni Yoga

Agni Yoga is a synthesis of all yogas, especially Karma Yoga, Bhakti Yoga and Raja Yoga. Agni is the Sanskrit word for Fire – the Creative Fire of the Cosmos, the fire that is found in varying degrees at the foundation of all Yogas.

Mantra Yoga

Mantra Yoga allows the practitioner to find union with God through the proper use of speech and sound. It is the power of the word to create or destroy that Mantra Yoga emphasises. It utilises the focus intent to make every word you speak be in harmony with God and with your own soul.

Yantra Yoga

Yantra Yoga is the path of union with God thorough geometric visualisation. A yantra is a geometric design. They are highly efficient tools for contemplation, concentration, and meditation.

Sapta Yoga

Sapta Yoga is based on the ancient Yogic text, the *Gheranda Samhita*. It is both a spiritual practice and a therapeutic art and is successful in removing the causes of numerous diseases highly resistant to orthodox Western healing methods

Ashtanga Yoga

As previously discussed, yoga is basically a philosophy of life, which also has the potential to create a vibrantly healthy body and mind.

Ashtanga yoga is a more energetic form of the traditional practice of yoga. When it is practised in its correct sequential order, it gradually leads the practitioner to rediscovering his or her fullest potential on all levels of human consciousness – on physical, psychological, and spiritual levels. Through this practice of combining the correct breathing (Ujjayi Pranayama), postures (asanas), and gazing points (driste), the practitioner will be more able to gain control of his or her senses and will discover a very deep awareness of his or herself. By maintaining this discipline regularly and with great devotion, it is possible to acquire perfect steadiness of body and mind.

The word Ashtanga literally means eight limbs,

again coming from the Sanskrit language. These eight limbs with regard to Ashtanga specifically are described by Patanjali as Yama (abstinences), Niyama (observances), Asana (postures), Pranayama (breath control), Pratyahara (sense withdrawal), Dharana (concentration), Dhyana (meditation), and Samadhi (contemplation). These branches all support and combine with each other. In other words, Asana practice must be established for proper practice of pranayama and is a key to the development of the yamas and niyamas. Once these four externally oriented limbs are firmly rooted, the last four internally oriented limbs will spontaneously evolve over time, with practice.

Vinyasa means breath-synchronised movement. The breath is the heart of this discipline and links asana to asana in a precise order. By synchronising movement with breathing and practising Mula and Uddiyana Bandhas (locks), an intense internal heat is produced. This heat helps to purify muscles and organs and will expel any unwanted toxins as well as releasing beneficial hormones and minerals, which can nourish the body when the sweat is massaged back into the skin. The breath regulates the vinyasa and ensures efficient circulation of blood. The result is a light, strong body.

There are three groups of sequences in the Ashtanga system. The Primary Series (Yoga Chikitsa) detoxifies and aligns the body. The Intermediate

Series (Nadi Shodhana) purifies the nervous system by opening and clearing the energy channels. The Advanced Series A, B, C, and D (known as Sthira Bhaga) integrate the strength and grace of the practice, requiring higher levels of flexibility and humility.

Each level must be fully developed before proceeding to the next, and the sequential order of asanas is to be meticulously followed. Each posture is a preparation for the next, developing the strength and balance required to move further in the sequence and practice.

Breathing in Ashtanga Yoga

As with all forms of yoga, the continuity of deep, even breathing cannot be overemphasised in the Ashtanga Yoga system. When breath feeds action, and action feeds posture, each movement becomes gentle, precise, and perfectly steady.

According to the teachings of Sri T. Krishnamacharya and Sri K. Pattabhi Jois, two well-respected Yogis, *Breath is Life*. Breathing is our most fundamental and vital act, no matter what the circumstances, and holds a divine essence – exhalation is seen to be a movement towards God, and inhalation is said to be an inspiration *from* God. This theory can be supported by the fact that our very last action in life is to exhale, which, in essence, is the final and total surrender to God.

Practising Ashtanga Yoga

It is said with most things that where there is no effort there is no benefit. Strength, stamina and sweat are unique aspects of this traditional Yoga, seemingly contrary to Western perceptions of Yoga. This demanding practice requires a great deal of effort and it taps into and circulates a vital energy throughout the body, strengthening and purifying the nervous system. The mind then becomes aware, clear and precise, and according to Sri K. Pattabhi Jois, "Wherever you look you will see God."

The use of meditation with Ashtanga Yoga

Although it is not is not necessary to practice yoga to meditate, it is true to say that meditation is an integral part of yoga. There are a great many techniques of meditation. The goal of meditation is enlightenment. The different approaches will all have the effect of quietening the mind even if the goal is not the objective. In yoga the process itself leads you to the point where meditation becomes the natural next step. There is no better antidote for the stress of modern living than meditation. If you are not exactly sure what meditation is, in its most simplistic form it is a method of switching off. It is a way of redirecting the activity or energies of the mind. At its highest it is transcendence – the experience of the unity of all life, the direct experience of who and what you really are, beyond form and limitation, Atman.

Bhuddist monks teach various techniques of meditation. These are mainly focused on working with the breath. The most basic is to observe the breath entering and leaving the nostrils. You will find that the mind will constantly wander away but with repeated practise will gradually stay focused. Another technique involves using the movement of the mind. By watching, and counting the incoming breath up to ten and on the out breath thinking of word which reflects a quality you wish strengthen in you character. On reaching ten count back to one, repeat the whole process a minimum of four times. Should you loose count start again from the beginning. Other techniques involve the use of mantra, which is discussed in greater detail through this book. The Sunlun techniques and mantra can lead to a completely altered state of consciousness.

CHAPTER 2
Before you start

When talking about the practice of Yoga, it is also
important to consider our eating habits and diet
which are by no means ideal. We all eat too quickly
and consume a lot of convenience food which are
obviously lacking in goodness. If you understand that
the purpose of eating is to supply our being with life-
force or prana then we can see that the best
nutritional plan is a diet of fresh, natural foods which
do not contain harmful additives. We should also eat
in a calm, relaxed atmosphere and chew food
thoroughly, as digestion actually begins in the mouth.
It is easy for us all to make excuses about not having
enough time for regular exercise but it only requires
about 15–20 minutes a day . The best times for
practising yoga are either first thing in the morning
,as this makes you more able to cope with any
problems that the day might bring, or last thing at
night which will help to promote a peaceful nights
sleep ensuring that you awake more refreshed. A few

simple breathing exercises practised at lunch time can give an energy boost for the rest of the day. Although Yoga can be practised by people of most ages and most physical abilities, it is advisable to check with a doctor before undertaking any programme of regular exercise. It is important to find a qualified teacher in your area who will be able to give you the correct advice for practice. Most areas run evening classes at their local colleges of education.

Why do people learn yoga?

There are many reasons why people in the West, who
do not come from a Hindu tradition and are
unfamiliar with the spiritual background of yoga, are
attracted to it and want to learn a little bit about it.

Some people are concerned with it only as a form
of exercise. Yoga strengthens the body, in particular
the spine, and develops suppleness and flexibility. A
stiff body not only feels uncomfortable, it is also
ageing. Even quite elderly people can move and walk
like those a third of their age if they remain supple
and lithe, and yoga helps achieve that. My first yoga
teacher was a woman who must have been in her 60s,
and yet if you saw her from a distance you would
have thought this was a young woman, such was her
lightness and ease of movement and the spring in her
step.

Regular yoga practice also tones and firms the
body, essential requirements for a youthful or healthy
appearance. This has nothing to do with body size.
However big you are, you can still be firm and toned,
and however slender you may be, unless there is
muscle tone you won't look lithe.

Sports by their very nature are competitive, with
winners and losers. In yoga there is no competition,
no 'best' or 'worst', no winners or losers. By learning
to perform a series of movements (the asanas)
individuals instead develop their own bodies, but the

emphasis is very much on the individual and his or her experience of his or her own body.

Health benefits

If you are suffering from any minor ailment (such as a sprain or a headache) or you are menstruating, you should inform the teacher before you begin practising yoga. If your problem is more serious or you are pregnant, you must inform your GP before starting any classes. This is for your own safety.

Regular classes are not suitable for those with certain medical conditions. Please inform your doctor and your teacher *before* starting classes if you have any of the following conditions: heart disease or any heart problem, epilepsy including petit mal, cancer or benign tumours, diabetes, meniere's disease, detached retina, AIDS, MS (multiple sclerosis) or if you have recently had an operation.

Having any of these conditions does not mean that you cannot practise yoga or that it will not be able to help you – on the contrary. It is simply best to go for the safety option, rather than risking your health and having to suffer the consequences. There will very probably be a remedial class at the centre you decide to use which will usually accept students with arthritis, asthma, back problems, diabetes, hernia, high blood pressure, knee problems, neck and shoulder problems, ME (myalgic encephalomyelitis), sciatica, whiplash. If you are in any doubt or have any concerns about your ability to do yoga, always contact your doctor.

Yoga therapy is the adaptation of yoga for people with health problems. Although general yoga classes can improve general health and resolve mild complaints, they may be ineffective – or even harmful – for serious conditions. In such cases, yoga therapy can help people by tailoring yoga to their individual needs, taking into account their health problems, constitution and circumstances. Yoga therapy uses the traditional practises from India, which date back thousands of years and were part of their traditional health care system. These practices are among the most effective known methods for managing stress-related conditions, which are so common today. This is because they bridge the gap between body and mind.

Many health benefits are claimed for yoga, and not the least of these is the overall sense of wellbeing and tranquillity that comes with regular practice.

The postures of yoga stretch the muscles and release the tension that is held within them; the lungs and chest are 'opened'; deep nasal breathing is an integral part of every session; and the spine – consisting of those 33 vertebrae that wrap around the spinal cord which has been described as the 'information superhighway of the body', transmitting sense and meaning directly to the 'central computer' of the brain – is strengthened.

Because of its calming and relaxing aspects, anyone suffering from stress or a stress-related disorder will benefit from yoga. The list of ailments for which people claim relief through yoga is long and varied, and these are only a few of them:

- Insomnia
- Anxiety and/or depression
- Sinusitis
- Hypertension
- Digestive disorders
- Pre-menstrual tension and painful periods
- Backache

As well as allowing us a calmer frame of mind, yoga builds strength and suppleness in the body, and a supple body remains youthful and active. It is therefore much recommended for older people. After the menopause women are more prone to brittle-bone disease (osteoporosis) as hormonal changes lower the body's calcium levels and the mineral content of the bones; strengthening the muscles which protect the skeleton and stretching and flexing the spine can help prevent that muscle-wastage and physical frailty that puts older people at risk of broken bones.

If you go into a bookshop, or search any of the online Internet stores such as Amazon, searching for titles on yoga, you will find among many many others books with the following special relevance: Yoga in Pregnancy, Yoga for the Menopause, Yoga for Women, The Yoga Back Book, Yoga for Pain Relief, Yoga at your Desk – the list goes on.

Interest in alternative or complementary therapies has increased noticeably in recent years, and a growing number of people daily seek professional help from practitioners of aromatherapy, acupuncture, homeopathy, reflexology and herbal medicine, to name but a few. Yoga belongs very firmly within that structure, not because it offers specific remedies for particular ailments – it is not a medical treatment – but because it belongs in a tradition both of holistic and preventative medicine.

The holistic tradition believes that mind and body are one, and that in treating an ailment the whole person must be treated, rather than just the ailment. Conventional Western medicine has tended to regard a disease or condition as if it was somehow separate from the human being that has it. A person suffering from, say, a digestive disorder, will be given medication or, drastically, surgery that is concerned only with suppressing the symptoms and removing the malignancy of that condition. A holistic practitioner starts from who the person is, asking for a detailed history of their lifestyle, state of mind and daily habits, believing that the origins of the disease or condition will be found there. Take for example the case of someone in a highly stressful job leading a high-octane life – travel, long hours of work, pressure at work, rushed meals of fast food, alcohol for stimulation and 'relaxation', perhaps cigarettes as well – who develops an ulcer. Conventional medicine would prescribe drugs to treat the ulcer; holistic medicine would recommend a change of lifestyle and re-ordered priorities – good food, good rest, a minimum of alcoholic stimulation, a more tranquil approach – in order not only to cure the ulcer but to prevent its recurrence; it's not just the disease that needs healing, but the person who has the ailment.

At the heart of the philosophy of yoga is a belief in balance. Not just the balance of the body – achieving poise and grace through controlled postures – but the balance of the mind, too. Many Eastern religions and philosophies have at their core a belief in the existence of opposites in a cycle of conflict with each other: yin and yang, light and dark, heat and cold, death and birth, good and bad. The tension between opposites is necessary for life, is indeed the essence of life: but the balance between the two must be maintained in harmony. Chaos and disorder follow when the balance is lost.

In our own lives, too, we know that a certain amount of stress or tension is both unavoidable and necessary. The right amount of 'stress' – wanting to achieve, to do well, to pass an exam, to learn a new skill – drives us forward in a positive, challenging way. It is only when that stress becomes too much or is unreasonable or negative in origin (wanting to earn more money than other people, competing in an unhealthy way, working overly hard in a critical or negative environment) that our mental and physical health begins to deteriorate.

The practice of yoga teaches us that mind and body are one, and that when the body is relaxed and strong and supple so will the mind be also. It is impossible to practice yoga while feeling angry, tense or distressed. You might bring these emotions to a session, but once you start to breathe deeply and focus on the asanas such negativity dissolves and the mind is released from the prison of these feelings.

If you do have any existing health problems such as diabetes or hypertension or physical conditions (such as a bad back, or knee or joint problems), make sure you mention these to your teacher if you attend a yoga class. They won't stop you from doing yoga, but extra care has to be taken, and strength built up slowly. Your teacher may also teach you which particular asanas benefit those with your condition. If you are studying alone at home, give yourself extra time and leeway.

One of the major problems of today's stressful lifestyles and jobs is that of stress, depression, and more commonly insomnia, or lack of sleep. Insomnia can happen even if you are feeling very sleepy or physically tired. Often, the situation arises where you desperately need to sleep so that you will be properly rested and alert for going to work, or for a big night out, but you simply end up staring wide eyed at the bedroom ceiling. It can happen to anyone, even those who are usually heavy sleepers and have never had problems with sleep in the past. The symptoms are that your mind is overactive and agitated, and your body won't relax no matter how hard you try to relax and sleep. The harder you work at getting to sleep, the wider awake you end up becoming. Even if you try all of the traditional methods of getting to sleep, such as counting sheep, having a hot milky drink, having a quick snack, having some light exercise, they will generally be of very little success.

We have probably all experienced some form of insomnia at particularly stressful times in our lives. It is very normal to have trouble sleeping at these times, but the difference is that it usually passes after a night or two. Insomnia only becomes a major problem when it becomes chronic. Although the problem is associated with certain physical illnesses, such as arthritis, heart failure, and chronic lung disease, most experts agree that insomnia is a symptom of a problem and not an illness in itself.

Stress is one of the mental problems where yoga can be helpful. We all need a certain amount of stress in our lives to give us motivation and encouragement to continue, but when it restricts our daily life to a great extent, it can become a major problem and will begin to affect our health. We are all very different individuals and what may be regarded as a positive stress for one person might have a very negative effect on another. It is important, therefore, that we can learn to recognise our own capabilities and find some ways of managing any of the stressful events in our lives. It is not always possible or practical to avoid some of the situations that can cause the stress, so we have to find an effective way of assisting our selves to cope with the situation. It is important that we should all learn to take responsibility for our own health and bodies, and Yoga is one way of achieving this – the vast numbers of people who now practice the art of yoga means that something must be working for them! Yoga asanas are particularly helpful in relation to stress as they have a profound effect on our whole mind and body. Our central nervous system is nourished by the spine, and the condition of our spine is largely responsible for our physical and emotional well being. In Yoga practice, the spine is the most exercised part of the body so it is easy to see what the benefits of Yoga practice may be. Yoga postures also help to stimulate the lymphatic system that will help to remove toxins from the body that, if allowed to accumulate, will no doubt cause much pain and stiffness in the muscles and joints. The functioning of the glands is also regulated, which will create the correct balance in our system.

The spiritual dimension

In modern Western society, we tend to look outside ourselves for our happiness and wellbeing. Fulfilment is 'out there' – in money, in careers, in a busy social life, in holidays and clothes and material possessions. If we buy or acquire all of these, we will be happy. Even family and friends, although precious and a source of joy in our lives, are still 'out there', independent separate beings whose lives we do not control. In trusting material possessions or other people to make you happy, you are placing yourself in an emotionally vulnerable position. Money can vanish, and jobs be lost; human beings we depend on can die, or change, or simply go away and not want to be with us any more. The world then seems a cold and empty place, and we feel like lost and frightened children, crying for our mothers in the dark.

The philosophy of yoga allows us to look within ourselves, and to understand that the one certainty we have in life is the reality of ourselves. A self-sufficiency develops that allows love without dependence and 'possession' without fear of loss, because the only thing we truly own is ourselves.

Many people who come to yoga simply for the physical exercise are surprised to find themselves attracted to its spiritual dimension, while many people step on the yoga path in the first place because of its philosophy.

Those of us who live in the so-called 'First World' of the rich Western nations may be materially fortunate, but have come to realise that possessions and a healthy bank balance are not enough: of themselves, they don't bring happiness. 'Happiness' seems like an elusive butterfly we chase helplessly, always thinking we're just about to get it: the next job, the next relationship, the next holiday, the next shopping expedition – that will be it, we'll have 'caught' happiness. Instead, happiness flutters away from our grasp, yet again.

In yoga, the emphasis is not on 'out there', not on the future or the past, but on now. We learn to enjoy the present moment, the feeling of being alive and in our bodies at this very second.

Happiness is found in stillness, silence and inner peace. Our world is a very noisy place and many people are never alone and never quiet. It's almost as if we distrust or fear silence. Even people who do live alone rush to turn on the TV, the sound system or the radio as soon as they enter the front door, to smother the silence with a blanket of noise.

In order to practice yoga, you have to learn to be still and quiet, free of noise and distraction. For many people that alone is an unusual and rewarding experience. Until we sink into the peace of silence we often don't realise how exhausting noise is: the ceaseless hum of traffic, the loud, forced voices from the TV and the radio and the canned music in shops and pubs are as much a pollutant as petrol fumes or acid rain.

An image to hold in your mind is that of a wheel, or circle. In our Western philosophies we tend to think of life, or the passage of time, as a path or road. You get on the road at one point, travel to a destination, and when you die you simply leave – as if it's time for your motorway exit. There is a start point and a finish point. The Eastern philosophies of which yoga is a part see life in the image of a wheel: an endless cycle of death and rebirth, destruction and renewal. We always return to the same place. You can come home again, and do it better. In yoga the same postures are repeated again and again and again, but each repetition brings a new insight, a refreshment of the spirit.

The poet T. S. Eliot wrote:

> *We shall not cease from exploration*
> *And the end of all our exploring*
> *Will be to arrive where we started*
> *And know the place for the first time.*

Patanjali – The father of all types of Yoga

According to historical texts and traditions, the sage Patanjali lived in India approximately 2,200 years ago, sometime around 220 BC. It is said that he is the incarnation of the serpent Ananta, upon whom the Lord Vishnu rested before the beginning of creation. He was both a scholar and a philosopher, and the author of many classical treatises on yoga philosophy, Sanskrit grammar and medicine.

In the Yoga Sutras, Patanjali collated and organised all knowledge on the age old subject of yoga and, as a consequence, has come to be known as the 'father of yoga'. He demonstrated a profound understanding of human nature and psychology, and through this knowledge he leads the reader through a mental and spiritual evolution along the yogic path. In total, Patanjali codified the entire yoga system into 196 sutras.

Patanjali was also responsible for writing a classical commentary on grammar – known as the Mahabhasya – which was used to expand the knowledge of Sanskrit grammar by redefining its rules and enlarging its vocabulary with the aim of making the language fit for the finest of human thoughts.

Patanjali also commented on the ancient system of good health and life, Ayurvedic medicine. In particular, he focused on the formation and structure of the human body, the beauty and problems of the body, the diagnosis of diseases and the curative effects of pharmacological techniques.

In Indian iconography – the worshipping of icons in a religious way – Patanjali is often depicted as half human and half serpent, the man's torso extending from a base of serpent coils. His hands are usually shown in namaste, which is to indicate a meditative state and suggests that he is greeting and blessing us in our yoga practice. Two additional hands hold a conch shell that calls the student to practice, and a disc that represents the wheel of time and the law of cause and effect.

The use of herbs alongside yoga

Herbs have been used historically to heal the ills of human and animals. In Ayurvedic medicine (the earliest form of healing) herbs are one of a twenty-point plan for total health. Many pharmacological preparations come from or copy herbs. Unlike herbs, such preparations have side effects and – in excess – can actually cause death. Herbs have fewer or no known side effects. Herbs are not a quick fix, but provide food for the body systems, which may be lacking in the food we eat.

Herbs bring new health to the lives of many people. Their value as a medicine has been known for centuries. Herbal remedies were the natural drugs used to cure various ailments of long ago. King Solomon used herbs. Numerous references to herbs throughout the bible indicate that kings and commoners used herbs. Today's health conscious public is now realising that herbs can also bring all round better living. Athletes are finding that certain herbs give added strength and stamina. Herbs are helping thousands to control weight and keep in shape. As a beauty aid they far surpass any of the concoctions of today's cosmetologists. Students are finding that herbs enhance their alertness and mental capacity. Is it any wonder? Good health comes from good food, adequate exercise, and from giving special attention to particular areas of concern. With health as our goal and proper nutrition as our tool, we can bring a healthy balance to our lives. At the end of this section can be found a short list of some traditional remedies that have successfully been used to treat common health problems. They are not the only remedies, but serve as a guide to help people return to a state of good health. Herbs are the cleansers of the body, feeders of the glands and balancers of hormones. From our food, we should get our proteins, carbohydrates, fats, vitamins and minerals that rebuild and maintain our body. In today's society with its fast food, junk food and processed food many people are actually suffering from malnutrition and the supermarket shelves are often stocked with de-vitalised and poor nutrition goods. In the natural process of functioning, the body produces toxic substances, which it cannot always eliminate and which build up in the body, this creates a toxic condition, which undermines health. Herbs enable the body to function more efficiently by removing the toxins. When herbs are used to restore health the dosage will need to be five to seven times the dose required to maintain health. Depending of course on the ailment and its severity, a sustained high dosage of approximately 3 months is usually required before the body is returned to health. Sometimes it may take a full year for reparation to occur so that a person goes through all four seasons. The science of Homeopathy teaches that it takes one month for every year of illness for the person to rebuild the body. Medical science has rightly made us aware of the dangers of overdoses and wrong dosages. With herbs you can set the mind at rest. Herbs are food not drugs. If taking medication in addition to herbs, advice should be sought from the company. Herbs are not a quick fix. Years of neglect or misuse, will not be repaired overnight. Herbs should be given a fair chance. Allow your body to heal slowly, naturally and effectively with herbs. There are few precautions with regard to taking herbs and if in any doubt seek advice from your health care professional. Most herbs can be taken throughout pregnancy with no ill effects, indeed many are positively beneficial just before childbirth. Some herbs however are contra indicated during pregnancy (most companies state so when this applies). Children can safely use herbs, however the dosage would have to be adjusted according to age, size etc. Should there be any doubt seek further advice. Many herbalists advocate the use of nutrient herbs throughout the growing years to build strong healthy bodies.

Statistics for the USA for the period 1983–1992 show that:

    320 deaths caused by over-the-counter drugs
    9000 deaths caused by food borne illness
    Deaths caused by herbs – zero

Figures for the UK are no less alarming and
statistics from the Department of Health state that:
In the UK 1.7 million patients are admitted to
hospital each year because of illness caused by
doctors or their treatment

How do I start my study of yoga?

Often, when beginning to study the art of yoga, people like to begin with the Om Chanting Technique. This technique is used as a form of meditation in yoga, and is a good starting point, so that you can relax your body and mind before trying any yoga positions. It is also a way to begin to focus your mind and your energies, which will become more and more important as you become more expert in the art.

To undertake the technique of om chanting, you should begin by sitting in the Sukhaasan or lotus position – or any comfortable posture which allows your spine to be erect. After you are in this position, close your eyes. You should then allow your shoulders and neck to relax completely, without relaxing and bending your spine. Allow all of your thoughts to settle and slow down completely. At this point it is important to consciously watch your breathing for a few moments – you should pay particularly close attention to your exhalation, and the little pause at the end of the exhalation. This pause is said to be a mystical moment before you draw in your next breath. You should also try to sense the stillness in your body and mind. Try to focus and sense the quietness of your breath. Also observe the associated calmness of your mind.

Now, use all your energies and focus to inhale

mindfully, and, as you exhale, you should make the sound of the the mantra "OM", smoothly and clearly. It is best to do this on your own for at least the first few times, as you may be a bit uptight if someone is witnessing you doing this. The duration of your OM chanting should always be as long as the duration of your exhalation. Do not try to stretch the sound beyond the exhalation and make your self short of breath. In other words, allow the chant to last *only* as long as your exhalation. At this point of the practice, you should attempt to pay attention to the resonance of this powerful mantra and notice how the whole body and mind respond to the OM chant.

This whole process should be repeated a second and third time. Watch how the last OM tapers into inner silence. This silence should be relished and enjoyed for a few moments – you have obtained inner peace.

Now, bring the attention back to the breath and again observe – or, at least, notice – the stillness of the breath. It is important to savour the effect of the chant for as long as you like, with eyes closed.

The practice of om chanting improves each time you undertake it. You may have thought it was simply a case of sitting with your spine upright, chanting and making funny noises! But, with practice, you will be able to see and to appreciate the immense effect it can have on your body and mind. When your body, mind and spirit are in union and in harmony, our daily lives will be affected for the better. Life's challenges will become less of a bind and we will begin to see them as factors that can only enhance our lives and mature well.

Learning Yoga itself

Yoga is believed to be about 6000 years old, originating in India. However there are several sources claiming it to be considerably older. Yoga is a dynamic system of physical exercise and a valuable philosophy to apply to everyday life. The ultimate goal of yoga philosophy is complete detachment from reality, as we understand it, and complete self knowledge or Samadhi. Only by separating 'self' from our environment can we come to terms with individual personality and start putting the mind and emotions in order. This lack of self knowledge is thought to be the fundamental cause of many emotional and nervous problems. The word YOGA comes from Sanskrit language and means union. There are various Yoga systems but the goal is always the same, which as we have said, is perfect self knowledge. The most popular form of Yoga practised in this country is Hatha yoga that is concerned with body control and consists of a series of exercises or asanas.

The word HATHA is made up of HA meaning sun and THA meaning moon. The body is enlivened by positive and negative currents and when these are in complete equilibrium we enjoy perfect health. Although Hatha yoga is essentially concerned with control of the body it has a much wider effect as in a fit body all systems function efficiently which will in turn help to calm the mind. About 2500 years ago

Buddha stated "you are what you think " and Patnajali considered to be the father of traditional yoga defined yoga as controlling the activities of the mind. Most exercise programmes depend mainly on working on the body ignoring the fact that the body and mind have a great effect on each other. Yoga is one of the concepts that could today be described as holistic or in other words affecting the body, mind and spirit i.e. the 'whole' person. Yoga helps people to take control of their lives by learning to control the body, breath and mind. The secret is to find a balance in life. It has been said that yoga is not for one who eats too much or too little, not for one who sleeps too much or too little the idea is to achieve moderation in all aspects of ones life.

The best way of learning yoga is to find a teacher whom you like and attend classes. Most sports centres and yoga centres allow you the chance to go along and join in a couple of classes and pay for them individually, without committing to paying for a whole course or series of classes. It is always recommended, with any sport or art, that you should attend a certified class, rather than simply learning from a book or manual. This is because the class will be instructed by a proper teacher and will encourage you to get the best out of yourself and will motivate you to do so. The other reason is for safety. With all sports and physical activities – including yoga – there is always the chance of incurring a personal injury or muscle strain, and an instructor will either be trained to assist with this or there will be first aiders within the centre. Another benefit of a teacher is that he or she can correct your postures and prevent you getting into 'bad' habits in the asanas that might be harmful. For instance, resting on the back of your head rather than the crown in the Fish pose, or tensing the neck or shoulders in another pose.

Yoga is now so popular that in some areas there is even a shortage of teachers to cope with the demand from the public. In large cities or urban areas you will find a choice of classes, whereas in less populated areas you may only have a choice of one that will be able to take you. You will probably only be able to attend a class once a week, but in between times you can obviously use a book such as this one to practice on your own at home.

To give some advice on home practice, it has been said that the art of practice is about knowing what to do, when to do it and how much of it to do. To sum this up with regard to yoga, yoga is not too much, not too little, not too early, not too late. Obviously, there will be people reading this who are at a different stage in developing their practice of yoga, but the rules are basically the same for us all.

Classes vary enormously – in size, in the age and sex of students and in focus. Some classes concentrate solely on the postures of yoga, while other teachers include periods of meditation in their classes, others focus on relaxation techniques and read passages on the philosophy of yoga. You may decide that you would prefer to practice in your own way alone at home, but as with all sports or physical activities it is difficult, however brilliantly a book may be illustrated or a video presented, to see exactly how something is done from that source alone.

In many areas of the country, there is also the possibility of attending yoga workshops. These are usually held at weekends and consist of one- or two day-courses. These are a wonderful way of getting started and to see what the art of yoga may be able to offer you, and will offer others the opportunity to spend an extended, intensive period of time immersed in yoga practice.

You should check your usual local information sources – the library, local directories, local news papers, notice boards in health food stores, adult education departments at schools and universities – to find out what is available near you. If you have access to the Internet and search for information on yoga, you will find yourself bombarded with a wealth of web sites you can visit.

A list of addresses is given at the end of this book.

What do I need?

If you are attending a yoga class, all you will need are loose-fitting clothes which you can move around comfortably in. There are of course various leotards and 'yoga wear' available for those who want to buy them, but they are not necessary to benefit from the art. Many people just wear a cotton T-shirt and jogging trousers or leggings. Make sure you can move your arms freely, and bend your legs without restriction (in other words, don't wear jeans!). Very loose-fitting T-shirts or those with low necklines can be a nuisance if they fall over your head when you bend over.

Yoga should always be practised in bare feet. However, many community halls or school gyms (the sort of places where classes are held) can be quite chilly and you should take socks and a sweatshirt to put on for the relaxation or meditation periods when you won't be moving and stretching and keeping warm. It will obviously be impossible to relax if you're shivering an uncomfortable.

As there is a lot of stretching and bending involved in the practice of yoga, women should also consider the kind of bra they are wearing. There's nothing more irritating and un-conducive to concentrated calm than sliding straps that have to be repeatedly hauled back up. Special sports bras or dance tops can be helpful for this reason.

Remove your watch: your teacher will know how the time is going, and if you are alone at home, learn to trust yourself to know when you have done enough. Also, for comfort and safety, remove dangling earrings, necklaces, etc.

Most classes make floor mats available for students, but it is often best to acquire your own, as cushioned exercise mats are seldom big enough and often slide about on polished floors. Specialist yoga mats are not only long enough to lie down on, but are made of a non-slip material. Such mats can be bought from various yoga organisations, including the British Wheel of Yoga (address at the end), but class teachers often arrange to bulk-purchase these for their students.

Your teacher should also provide a foam or sponge block if you need one. There are small rectangular blocks that can help those who have knee or back problems, or beginners who are finding some of the poses challenging. Many people, for instance, find it uncomfortable to sit cross-legged, and one of these blocks under the buttocks helps. Others can't sit on their knees, but can do so with a foam block slipped under the buttocks and cushioning the heels. If you have neck problems, you may find it helps to slip one under your neck for extra support when lying down.

If you are practising at home you can buy one of these foam blocks yourself, from the British Wheel of Yoga or another supplier, or simply use a small cushion or pillow for the same effect.

Yoga space at home

If you want to practice yoga at home, either in between classes or instead of classes, you need to set aside a space and a time for this.

Of course this does not need to be rigidly structured: as far as time is concerned, you need a minimum of 10–15 minutes when you are undisturbed, preferably longer, and a space in which you can lie down and raise your arms without bumping into furniture and hurting yourself.

A little structure does help, however, not least because it emphasises that this is your special time and your special space. The purpose of any kind of ritual is to heighten awareness and emphasise importance, and what you are doing – since it relates to your health and wellbeing – is very important.

If your bedroom or spare room has enough floor space, then that is ideal. The sitting room is fine, too, but remember that ground-floor rooms might be overlooked and nothing spoils the concentration quicker than an audience does!

Before you start your yoga session, switch on the answer phone and switch off the TV and the radio. If you live with other people, explain to them that you would like to be left alone for a while. Persuade the cat and the dog to leave you alone while you do your stretching exercises and shut them, temporarily, out of the space where you are.

Some people like to create a spiritual atmosphere with candles or incense while they practice. Anything that adds to your sense of calm, pleasure and purpose that is not a distraction (I trust you to know the difference) is good.

If you are learning yoga at home with a book, it is hard to read instructions while bending over backwards at the same time! It will take you a while to remember a posture, and so at the beginning there will be a lot of stopping and starting while you pick up the book again to check what you're doing. Don't worry about this, but do bear two things in mind.

1   When learning with a book, try just to concentrate on one posture at a time and 'learn it by heart'. If you are a complete beginner and attempt to read your way through four or five postures at once you may become frustrated and confused and give up altogether. It's best to decide to do just one thing (for example, the forward bend or the Dog) and become completely familiar with that asana before moving on.

2   If you have to keep referring to a book you will be going into and coming out of your posture. Take care not to strain yourself while doing so. If, for instance, you're resting on your elbows with your head back in the pose of the Fish and you forget what to do next, take care how you get up to check the book. At all times, come out of positions gradually, taking care to

'unroll' your spine or lift your head carefully.

If you have a friend who also wants to study yoga at home, this could work very well. You could check each other's postures – perhaps one reading from the book while the other assumes the pose – and give each other motivation and encouragement.

How long does a yoga session take?

Classes usually last an hour, which allows time to warm the muscles up at the beginning with some stretching postures, and often a period of relaxation at the end.

If you are practising at home, then of course it's up to you. Human nature being what it is, I know I would find it easier to set aside 10–15 minutes a day than tell myself I'll do a full hour on Sunday morning – somehow, that full hour would never arrive. And with all forms of physical exercise, little and often is better than quite a lot all at once and not very often. It is also true that when you are new to something, 15 minutes seems like a long time, but as you grow in experience and knowledge, it's hardly anything. As you become more flexible and supple, you will want to practice more.

If you are beginning, why not take one asana a day and work on that for 10 minutes? The following week, you could link two postures together and practice them, and so on. Spend one week concentrating on the Sun Salutation and learning that, so that you can integrate that into your daily practice. Some summer mornings, you might even want to get up early and really salute the sun as it rises.

What do I need to know?

In your yoga class, or in looking through yoga books
and videos, here are a few things you may come
across that may be unfamiliar to you, or that you may
have a question about.

Nemaste Some of the instructions below mention
'hands to nemaste'. Nemaste is the prayer position in
yoga. Place the palms together, as in prayer, and bring
your hands to the sternum – your breast-bone
(literally, the bony place you can feel between your
breasts). As with so much in yoga, nemaste has a
mind-and-body relevance. In bringing your hands to
nemaste, you remember the spiritual significance of
what you are doing. If you do not wish to be part of
this, just remember that the pose itself gives a good
stretch to the elbows, forearms and chest. If you pray
for nothing else, let nemaste acknowledge the wonder
of your body.

Loosen up At the end of strenuous cycles of yoga
(for example the Sun Salutation) always loosen up.
You will have worked your muscles hard, and they
need to be relaxed. This is not complicated. Simply
shake everything you can, as if you were a rag doll or
a puppet on strings that the puppeteer has dropped.
Rotate your shoulders, roll your head gently on your
neck, and shake your hands and feet as if they were a
bit loose and by shaking them you could drop them
off your arms and legs.

If you have been working your spine hard (for example in a Shoulder stand), or in any of the asanas that involves lying down (for instance the Fish) a helpful way of resting is to lie on your back and clasp your knees to your chest with your arms. Then gently rotate, clockwise and then anti-clockwise, as if you were an egg on a table. This roll helps rest a back that has been stretched.

Om is also sometimes spelled Aum. Many yoga classes begin and end with the class all sitting cross-legged, eyes closed, repeating Om 3 times. It is a Sanskrit word of very ancient origin meaning wholeness or 'one' – there is a link with the Greek letter omega, and just as in the Bible Jesus describes Himself as alpha and omega – the beginning and the end – Om is also taken to be a reference to the Creator. In repeating it, we put ourselves in touch with the Creator and with the spirit of creation. It is a mantra said to be older than time, reflecting the vibration of the universe and the breath of the Universal Being. When you intone Om, breathe in before you say the first letter and breathe out as you say the second, so that the sound of Om is as of a long release of breath, vibrating with the 'm'.

Chakras   The word chakra means wheel. In Eastern philosophy, the body contains a number of chakras (both major and minor ones) that may be defined as energy centres. The life force (prana, or chi) flows through them, connecting us to the world and to our own spirituality, directing movement and action. The major chakras are to be found in the crown of the head and at various points down the spinal column: behind the eyes at the top of the spine, the throat, the heart, the solar plexus, the sacrum and the coccyx at the base of the spine. It is believed that meditation, yoga and 'right living' keep these chakras clear and open; when chakras are 'blocked', the body becomes unbalanced and sickness of mind and body follows. Yogic asanas aim to keep the chakras flowing free and open.

Mudras The word mudra actually means a seal, and in yoga this refers to the posture of the hands in any asana. For instance, in alternate-nostril breathing (see below) the position of the hand and fingers in called the nadi-sodhana mudra. The one beginners most often encounter is the jnana mudra, used in many sitting postures. In this, the hands are rested lightly on the knee with the palms facing upwards and the index finger and thumb lightly touching. This represents the union of the individual soul with the life force.

Sitting cross-legged I mention this here because many people who think of yoga think at once of the Lotus position. In this, while sitting cross-legged, the left knee is bent as close to the body as possible while the right knee is tucked over the left, the foot being placed high up on the left thigh. As many people find sitting cross-legged at all uncomfortable, this puts

them off yoga before they've even started. As with
Shoulder stands (see below), don't worry if you can't
do it as it looks in some illustrated books. If you can
manage to sit in a simple cross-legged position, that's
fine. A foam block or cushion placed under the
buttocks can be an enormous help. If you have severe
problems with your knees, you may find you have to
sit with one or both knees out in front of you.
Generally, people find that as they practice and gain
flexibility, movements that once seemed out of the
question become comfortable and possible for longer
periods of time.

Before or after meals?

As with all forms of exercise, don't do yoga on a full
stomach – wait at least an hour after a heavy meal
and preferably two. On the other hand, if you're
stomach is completely empty you may find yourself
getting dizzy in some of the bending postures. The
approach is a 'suck it and see' one, and you will soon
find what works best for you.

Types of practice of yoga

Wit is possible to divide the practice of yoga up into three different types, depending on the interaction of the pupil and the teacher. The first type would be a class where the order of each asana and the time spent in each is given by a teacher. The second type is where the order and occasionally the time spent is given by a book or a sequence. The third is where the student is completely alone and must rely on his or her memory and creativity for the structure of the practice they carry out.

Our Changing State

It is a fact that the human body and its consciousness are always in a state of constant vibration. The correct and effective practice of asana and pranayama will serve to still this vibration and will take us to the state of union – yoga. Every day we are different and every moment we are different, therefore we must learn to tailor our practice to the needs of each of these moments. This is the art of practice.

It would be easy for you to simply say that on Mondays you will practise standing poses, then on Tuesdays you will focus on forward bends and so on. The problem with this way of looking at life is that we absolutely cannot predict our physical or mental state in advance at any time. Therefore to prescribe the method of practice before the moment could be like giving someone cough medicine to cure a broken leg. It may sound like an extreme way to describe it, but it is in no way an exaggeration.

External conditions must also be taken into account – for example, the temperature directly affects the elasticity and the flexibility of our muscles – and therefore care must be taken to ensure that on cold days there is adequate warm up. In very hot weather, fatigue will come about much more quickly, and thus more recuperative poses can be included.

Sequences of yoga

Sequences can become rituals and/or devotional acts that are to be done in a specific order, regardless of any external influences or the internal state. This enables one to begin to bring about a controlling of the consciousness, thus revealing an element of Bhakti Yoga in the sequences.

Sequences are a very useful tool for the beginner because they can be written down or remembered. So, instead of thinking of what you should be doing, you simply start at the beginning and carry on to the end without your mind wandering elsewhere.

It is also an advantage to use sequences because you are able to choose at the beginning of your practice which one of these sequences you will carry our, based on your condition, your time available and any other factors which may be restricting you, and the sequence can be adjusted or adapted in any way to suit these factors. Thus there is some creative input on the practitioner's part. For beginners, the teacher can be of great help at this stage, by suggesting various appropriate sequences. Reliance on sequences should lessen as you begin to advance along the yogic path and also as you begin to improvise your own sequences in response to the body-mind performance.

Groups of poses in yoga

Any person who is attending even just a few yoga classes will very soon realise that there is only a small number of groups that all poses can be put into, i.e. standings, sittings, supine, inverted, forward, back, twists and balancings. Each group can be characterised by the specific parts of the body that it works. Putting inappropriate emphasis on some of these groups will mean that the body begins to develop unevenly and there will be disharmony and conflict of emotion within the practitioner.

This might not show itself immediately, but nevertheless this issue should be addressed at every single practice session. You must strive to cover the main groups over a period of time. Classes could be organised around a monthly cycle. Standing poses in the first week, forward bends in the second week, backbends third week, recuperative poses and pranayama in the fourth week. Remember what was said earlier though – you cannot simply use each of these groups. There must be some sort of balance among the groups.

Ordering poses within a practice

This can be addressed at two levels. Firstly, at an over-all level, through the order of the groups, and secondly, at a much more subtle level, through the order <u>within</u> each of the groups. Certain groups of poses are appropriate for warming up (for example, at the beginning of the practice session) and others can be used for cooling down and relaxing at the end of each practice. There is a often a tendency within groups for the stretch or work to increase and deepen.

When you begin moving between two very different kinds of groups there are also transitional poses. For example there are many 'neutral poses'. That is to say that when you are moving from backward bends to forward bends, because the stretch is opposite, it is obvious to say that a neutral position is needed and is therefore evident right in the middle, just as when we are changing gear in a car we must move through the neutral position. One neutral gear for the above example is the use of gentle twists or for more advanced practitioners Bakasana. Also in a practice session, you may not be able to do a whole string of active poses without a break. An example of the use of neutral is Padottanasana. This position allows and provides a rest between the basic standing poses and the more demanding standing balances and standing twists.

Within groups of poses, the idea is to work from the most do-able position – not necessarily the easiest – to the least do-able. This is usually from a mild stretch to an intense stretch. For example, for a back bending sequence, do Supta Virasana, Ustrasana, Urdhva Dhanurasana and not vice versa.

Counter poses

Some schools of yoga have the practice of
constructing routines from pairs of poses. This is
where each pose is followed by a counter pose that
will allow the body to rebalance, for example
Matsyasana after Sarvangasana. In this type of yoga,
the emphasis is that the balance is achieved over the
whole session and not necessarily between two poses.

Towards difficult poses

For more advanced practitioners of yoga, one practice
session may not be long enough to build up to a
difficult posture and it may be more effective and
safer to build up over a period of days. This will
provide a much firmer foundation rather than being
over-ambitious. It may be worth undertaking an
intensive course of up to a few weeks long...

Motivation within the practice of yoga

Lack of motivation in any circumstance can mean
lack of energy. It is worthwhile to try resting poses or
energy-giving poses if you feel that you are lacking
the motivation necessary to practise yoga. Also it is
always worth trying a few poses even if you are a little
tired, because often the mind will quickly become
involved and interested in adjusting, reflecting and re-
adjusting, thus generating more ideas and energy for
practise. If nothing comes, try a different tack. This is
true in all areas of life – not just in the practice of
yoga itself.

Time OF day and times PER day

In the truest sense, yoga should be practised well
before dawn, then at midday, then just after dusk and
at midnight. In tropical countries, this conveniently
divides the long day into roughly equal quarters.
However, for the average practitioner, this is a bit
much and will be completely unrealistic if you have a
job – or a life at all! Practice generally happens
whenever it can be fitted in to today's busy lifestyle,
but there is also some room for making practice time
available. This will usually mean that compromises
will have to be made between practice, family, work,
eating, shopping and friends.

It is best to have a few hours that have been
completely food-free before practice. This obviously
means that post-waking, pre-breakfast is an ideal time
to practice. At this time of day, the mind should be
nicely rested but the body may well be a little stiff.
Another good time for practice is straight after work
and before dinner.

CHAPTER 3

An introduction to some basic yoga positions

Om Chanting Technique

This technique is used as a form of meditation in yoga, and is a good starting point, so that you can relax your body and mind before trying any yoga positions. It is also a way to begin to focus your mind and your energies, which will become more and more important as you become more expert in the art.

To undertake the technique of om chanting, you should begin by sitting in the Sukhaasan or lotus position – or any comfortable posture which allows your spine to be erect. After you are in this position, close your eyes. You should then allow your shoulders and neck to relax completely, without relaxing and bending your spine. Allow all of your thoughts to settle and slow down completely. At this point it is important to consciously watch your breathing for a few moments – you should pay particularly close attention to your exhalation, and the little pause at the end of the exhalation. This pause is said to be a mystical moment before you draw in your next breath. You should also try to sense the stillness in your body and mind. Try to focus and sense the quietness of your breath. Also observe the associated calmness of your mind.

Now, use all your energies and focus to inhale mindfully, and, as you exhale, you should make the sound of the the mantra "OM", smoothly and clearly. It is best to do this on your own for at least the first few times, as you may be a bit uptight if someone is witnessing you doing this. The duration of your OM chanting should always be as long as the duration of your exhalation. Do not try to stretch the sound beyond the exhalation and make your self short of breath. In other words, allow the chant to last *only* as long as your exhalation. At this point of the practice, you should attempt to pay attention to the resonance of this powerful mantra and notice how the whole body and mind respond to the OM chant.

This whole process should be repeated a second and third time. Watch how the last OM tapers into inner silence. This silence should be relished and enjoyed for a few moments – you have obtained inner peace.

Now, bring the attention back to the breath and again observe – or, at least, notice – the stillness of the breath. It is important to savour the effect of the chant for as long as you like, with eyes closed.

The practice of om chanting improves each time you undertake it. With practice, you will be able to see and to appreciate the immense effect it can have on your body and mind. When your body, mind and spirit are in union and in harmony, our daily lives will be affected for the better. Life's challenges will become less of a bind and we will begin to see them as factors that can only enhance our lives and mature well.

With the following positions and postures, please do not try any of these without reading at least the 'Before you start' chapter and remember the golden rule that yoga is a form of exercise meant to be practised and learned over many, many years. The more you do it, the more supple you become, so if you are unfit, or unused to exercise, or have been ill, then take things easily and gently to start with. You will gain nothing by hurting yourself and having to give up yoga altogether because of injury.

And – while this is undoubtedly stating the obvious, but we all forget it sometimes – remember that when you watch a yoga video, or a yoga teacher in action, or look at the illustrations in a big glossy yoga book – remember that the people who pose for these pictures are all very experienced yoga practitioners who have been repeating these poses for years and years. Almost certainly, you will not be able to achieve the same levels of stretch or balance or pose as they can; but that does not mean to say that you won't do so one day. Remember the wise saying:

"A journey of a thousand miles begins with a single step." Everything that you can do for yourself is important.

Some yoga books are very precise about the length of time for which you should hold certain postures – 3 minutes, 30 seconds, 45 seconds.

In describing the exercises below, I use the phrase: "Hold for as long as is comfortable".

For one thing, you should take off your watch when you practice yoga, and remove or ignore the clock if there is one in the room. Yoga practice is not about time, but about your time.

Second, once a posture becomes uncomfortable it is of no value to you.

Third, the length of time you can 'hold' a pose varies according to so many factors: your experience, your level of health or fitness, even the time of day. Even for experienced practitioners, there can be a world of difference between a posture that is assumed at 8 a.m. on a chilly morning, when you're cold and stiff from a night's sleep, and 8 p.m. in the evening, when the muscles are toned after a day's activity.

Yoga postures are not meant to be easy: you should feel a sense of stretch, of effort, of challenge. As in all forms of physical activity, you need to feel that you are working. That's the fun of it.

However, you should not be in pain. As has been said before, yoga (again, as with all physical activity) is cumulative: the more you do, the more you can do.

And there are levels in yoga, as in everything else. Just as you would not expect a 9-year-old attending Saturday dance classes to submit to the rigorous discipline of a morning session at the Royal Ballet, so you should not sign up for a yoga class and expect to hook your foot around your left ear in the first week. There are many, many yoga asanas left out of this book because they are impossible and daunting for beginners. If you continue your yoga practice, you will come to them when you are ready.

So if something hurts, stop doing it. The physical benefits of the yoga postures described below come from 'holding' that posture and making your muscles work, but you, and only you, know the difference between muscles being challenged and stretched and muscles just being hurt. Nourish that knowledge.

On a more practical level and for the purposes of this book I am assuming that 'Hold for as long as is comfortable' refers to a time that is between a few seconds and a few minutes. It may be that you have the willpower to hold, for example, the pose of the Fish for 2 hours and 22 seconds. The point is that after about 3 minutes of that time it is probably not doing you any good, and yoga is all about doing you good.

And –

- Don't forget to breathe! In the instructions given below, you are occasionally told when to breathe in and breathe out. In classical yoga, when and for how long you inhale and exhale is important but as a beginner don't worry about that as long as you keep breathing deeply and easily.

- After each exercise, loosen up. Do this just by shaking your body and limbs loosely, as if you were a rag doll.

Breathing

Where no specific instruction about inhaling or exhaling is given, as a rule of thumb, in the majority of asanas, the following is true:

- If you are moving or stretching backwards, breathe in.

- If you are moving or stretching forwards, breathe out.

Warming up: Standing

Yoga teaches us to do simple things, but to do them with concentration, and purpose, and a sense of being here now.

Stand with your feet slightly apart, so that your weight is distributed evenly on both feet and your body weight is over your feet. Pay attention to your feet: every part of your foot should be actively supporting your body – in other words, check you're not leaning backwards or forwards.

Let your arms hang loosely by your sides.

Your knees should be straight, but not rigid.

Breathe in, breathe out, through your nose. Keep your lips lightly together.

Look ahead: check that you are not holding your head too far back (your chin will be raised) nor too far down (you should be able to get your clenched fist comfortably between your chin and your chest, with a little room to spare).

The crown of your head is reaching up towards the sky: don't tense up, just feel the very top of your head reaching, reaching up to make you tall, and supple, and free.

Mentally think up and down your body: your face, your cheeks, your lips, your ears, your neck, your shoulders, your hands, the great muscles of the thighs, the knees, the calves, the feet, the toes.

As you think of each of these parts of your body, release them. In action, they move as one: as part of you and your body. But now, when you are still, you can think of them as individual parts, capable of individual movement, individual tension.

Breathe in, and with every breath you send out from your body exhale, expel, all that tension, all that fear, all that negative holding.

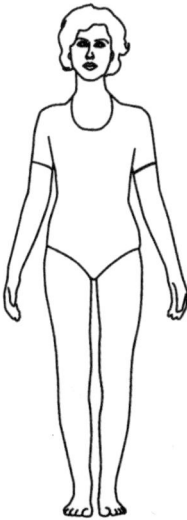

Warming up: Neck stretches

I   Sit cross-legged on the floor, in a position
     comfortable for you, with your back straight but
     not tense and your hands on your knees in the
     jnana mudra. This means that the tip of your
     index finger is touching the tip of your thumb
     making a circle, and the other fingers are fanned
     out naturally. Take a moment to sit with your eyes
     closed, breathing deeply and calmly.

     If you are aware of any tension in your body,
     let it go.

     Inhale, and move your head backwards. Don't
     'throw' your head back: make this slow movement
     last the length of your breath.

     Breathe normally. Check that your shoulders
     are relaxed.

     Breathe in again.

     Breathing out, move your head only (not your
     body) as far forward as you can. If you can, press
     your chin against your chest.

     Repeat this 2 or 3 times.

     What drives this movement is your neck, not
     your head or your chin. Think of your neck as a
     lovely, long flower on a stalk, bending backwards
     and forwards in the wind. The more your neck
     stretches itself, the longer and lovelier it will be.

     When you have finished, shake your shoulders
     and ease your head from side to side to loosen up.

2 With your eyes open, look straight ahead of you.
Keep your lips and mouth relaxed. Breathe in and
turn your face as far to the left as you can: it helps
to imagine that your eyes are following a beam of
light which moves right round to the left – but
only your head can move. Keep your shoulders
still.

Now follow that beam of light as it moves to
your right, as far as your neck can turn. Breathe
out.

Repeat this at least 2 or 3 times.

3 Eyes open, face forward, breathe in and tip your
left ear to your shoulder, breathing in. It helps to
imagine yourself lifting your head up by the
crown of the head before you tilt to the left. Keep
your shoulders still and down: don't bring them
up to meet your ear.

Breathe in, lift your head up; as you breathe
out, drop your right ear to your right shoulder.

Repeat this 2 or 3 times.

Variation I

As you tilt your head left and right, lift the opposite
shoulder. In other words:

Drop your head to the left, raise your right
shoulder (leave your arms loose and free).

Drop your head to the right, raise your left
shoulder.

Variation 2

Roll your head from side to side in one movement, on one breath. In other words: Breathe in, head to left shoulder, hold breath, head to right shoulder, free breath.

Warming up: Neck roll

Roll your head around on your neck. This time, imagine that your head is moving independently, as if it was a ball and your neck the "socket".

Start by taking a deep breath and lowering your chin on to your chest; free your breath as your chin drops down, then breathe again as you move your head in a circular motion to the left and then drop your head back, to the right and round again.

Repeat in the opposite direction. Keep your shoulders loose.

It's easy to feel dizzy if you do this too quickly.

You can do this position either sitting cross-legged or standing.

Shoulder exercises

I This is a soothing tension-buster. Do it sitting cross-legged on the floor, but it is the sort of exercise you can also do sitting at your desk or standing on the Tube (if you don't mind a few people giving you odd glances).

Then just rotate your shoulders in a circle, both together, first backwards 5 times, then forwards. Keep your head and your neck still, and try to imagine there is a pencil fixed to each shoulder, with which you are drawing a perfectly round circle.

2 Sitting cross-legged on the floor, bend your left elbow behind you and try to place your palm in the middle of your back. Now reach over your right shoulder with your right hand, and intertwine the fingers of both hands in the centre of your back. Breathing well, try to pull your hands apart, so that both elbows push away from each other in opposite directions.

Now bend forward as far as you can, while maintaining that hold between your hands.

Return to the upright, breathe, unlock your fingers and return your hands to your sides. Now repeat with the opposite arms.

Alternate-nostril breathing

Breathing is the essence of life, and of yoga.
Pranayama means breath control and comes from the
words prana, the life force (in this context breath
itself) and ayama – lengthening. Yoga aims to deepen
and lengthen the breath, just as if it were a muscle of
the body, and in doing so strengthens the life force
that is within each and every one of us.

We seek to exercise our bodies to make them
strong and supple, but should not neglect to 'exercise'
our breathing too, to make our capacity for breathing
strong and supple. At the core of most sports and
other forms of physical activity (dancing, swimming,
ballet, hill-walking, working out in the gym – even
just climbing the stairs) is the ability to breathe
properly: that is, taking breath into the abdomen (not
the chest) deeply and naturally, without strain. The
first thing singers are trained to do is breathe, and
classical singers are taught that unless and until they
can control their breathing effectively there is not
much point doing anything else.

People suffering stress often experience the
unpleasant sensation of a panic attack. The symptoms
of a panic attack are a tightening of the chest and
rapid, shallow breathing, accompanied by feelings of
acute fear and indeed panic – the symptoms so
resemble a heart attack that many people feel that's
just what they're experiencing. Deep breathing

overcomes such attacks and helps those suffering from stress.

The Nadi-Sodhana Mudra

In Sanskrit a mudra is a hand position (see the jnana mudra above) and this is the hand position for alternate-nostril breathing.

Sitting comfortably on the floor, preferably cross-legged if you can do this, close your eyes.

Leave one hand resting comfortably in your lap, and raise the other to your face. Place your index and middle fingers in the middle of your forehead, just above your nose.

Rest your thumb on your right nostril and your remaining two fingers – the third and little fingers – on the left nostril.

Gently 'close' your right nostril with your thumb, and breathe in deeply through your left nostril. Breathe as deeply as you can, as if you could blow away all the cobwebs in your brain by taking in this cleansing breath.

Now release your right nostril, and close your left nostril with the middle and little fingers together.

Breathe out through your right nostril.

Take breaths as deep as is comfortable, and hold them for as long as is comfortable. Concentrate on 'using' the nostril that is free for inhaling and exhaling, while keeping the opposite one gently closed.

The ha breath

This is a wonderful stress-buster.

Stand upright, legs slightly apart but parallel, and raise your arms above your head. Feel the stretch in your ribcage.

Bending from the hips, let the upper half of your body fall forward as if you are a puppet whose strings have suddenly been dropped. As you fall, deliberately say the word 'ha' as you propel the breath from your body. Allow your arms, head and upper body swing loose for a moment. Concentrate on forcing the breath from your lungs.

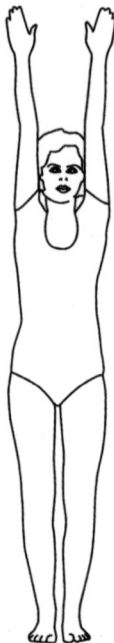

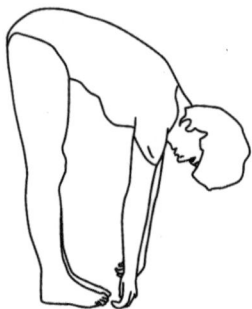

Be careful to come upright gently, without straining your back.

Kapalabhati (Cleansing breaths)

The aim of this is to clear the system and leave you feeling envigorated. You can practice it anywhere and in any situation where you need a boost of instant energy – for instance after lunch in the office, when we all feel sleepy at the prospect of the long afternoon ahead.

Sit cross-legged on the floor if you can, otherwise on a straight-backed chair.

The aim is to concentrate on inhaling and exhaling through the abdomen. As you do this, your diaphragm will rise and fall. Try to keep your shoulders and chest still: they are not involved in this process, although your chest will rise and fall naturally as your lungs fill and empty. The abdomen is the solar plexus, your tummy, the third chakra – it has been described as the psychic pump of the body.

To begin, pull in your tummy and breathe out: try to 'touch' your spine with your tummy as you do so. Automatically, your diaphragm moves up and your lungs empty.

Then relax: as you do so, your diaphragm will descend as you release your abdominal muscles and your lungs will open and take in air.

Repeat slowly, several times.

Try to visualise breathing as a process in which your whole body expands and contracts internally. Keep your mouth closed, but not tightly: in yoga, it is important to breathe through the nose.

The Lion

This asana tones the muscles of the face and neck, bringing them colour and firmness. It helps if you can lose your inhibitions and really make a face while you do it.

Sit cross-legged on the floor and spread your fingers open around your knees, as if you were covering the knee with a cloth. Then literally stick your tongue out: open your mouth wide, push your tongue out and down, and at the same time stretch your eyes open wide. Many people also like to make a deep growling noise at the same time! Think of it as if you are stretching every muscle of your face, just as you stretch your arms and legs in other exercises.

Stretching from a seated position

1   Sit cross-legged and relaxed, with your hands by
    your sides. Bring your palms together as in in
    prayer (nemaste, the prayer position) and slowly
    raise your arms above your head, breathing in.
    Stretched your arms straight above your head, as if
    your fingers could touch the ceiling.

     Face forward, and try to keep the rest of your
    body still. Reach with the crown of your head to
    lengthen your neck and your spine and help you
    with this reach, but your arms are doing the work:
    you should feel as if there is a thread attached to
    your fingertips which is pulling you up.

     Hold this position with your breath, and as
    you slowly lower your arms, breathe out.

     Repeat 2 or 3 times.

     Loosen up by rolling your shoulders back and
    round, as if you are trying to draw a circle with
    your shoulders.

2   Place your palms together and hold them to your
    chest, with the fingertips pointing outwards and
    the thumbs crossed, away from your body. Then
    stretch your arms straight out in front of you, as if
    you were diving slowly into a pool. Drop your
    chin on to your chest. Reach forward with your
    fingertips. Again, imagine that invisible thread
    attached to the very tips of your fingers, pulling
    you forward.

Breathe in, separate your palms and move your arms
behind you, keeping them at shoulder height.
Raise your head and look towards the ceiling (or
the sky, of course, if you are lucky enough to be
out of doors). The invisible thread is pulling your
arms behind you, like wings: feel a beneficial
stretch in your neck and shoulders.

Breathing out, swing your arms back again in front of
you, dropping your chin on to your chest, so that
you are back where you were before, 'diving' into
the air in front of you (but remember to keep your
arms up, at the height of your shoulders).

Repeat 2 or 3 times, concentrating on achieving a
good 'reach'.

3 Sitting cross-legged on the floor, raise your arms
to shoulder height on either side of you: your
palms should be facing down, and you are trying
to touch the wall on either side of you with your
fingertips. Try to visualise your armpits opening
and expanding, releasing your arms and allowing
them to reach that extra centimetre more. Your
spine is straight, your shoulders relaxed, not
tense. Keep breathing deeply: with each breath,
you will find your body gives you a little more
'reach'.

Be careful not to push your head forwards as
you try to achieve a better stretch. Your head
should remain balanced on your shoulders.

Maintaining this position, breathe in and twist your arms and your upper body to your left, keeping your head still but moving your eyes. When trying to achieve a good spinal twist, it is an idea to let your eyes 'lead you', as if there is something on the wall directly behind you that you are trying to see, but you can only move your body, not your neck alone. Hold this position and breathe out.

Breathe in again and swing round this time to the right. Hold this twist for a moment and then return to the centre.

Repeat several times, but in between each repetition pause and loosen up by shaking your arms free and rolling your shoulders. This process of loosening up will help you to achieve a better twist each time you do this.

4 Sitting upright, hold your elbows to your sides with your palms and forearms raised in front of you, as if you were carrying a light garment draped across both your arms in front. Don't stick your elbows out like teapot handles, keep them tucked in to your side.

Now pull your elbows back while raising your chin and dropping your head back. Feel as if you are trying to do two things: touch your back with the crown of your head, and touch your elbows behind your back. Even if you could, you should not actually do this of course! But try to feel the extension that you would have if you did this. Breathe well. If you feel tension bunching in your neck or your shoulders, release it.

Now bring your elbows forward and raise them in front of you, slowly dropping your chin on to your chest as you do so. With your head lowered, bring your arms together in front of your head so that your elbows are touching each other.

5 This is a more advanced stretch, and a variation on the spinal twist, so make sure you are fully warmed up before you do this.

Sit on your heels, with your back straight and your hands on your knees. As always, if sitting on your heels is not comfortable, try putting a cushion or a foam pad between your buttocks and your heels to pad them.

Now shift to your left hip and sit on the ground, so that your feet are now to the right, and your buttocks are to the left of where your feet are.

Raise your right knee and place the right foot flat on the floor. Your left leg will almost certainly have fallen to its side, so that your left foot is under your right buttock.

Now lift your right foot and place it outside on the ground outside the left thigh.

Your right hand is flat on the floor, palm

down, close to your right buttock.

Raise your left hand, and bring it over the right side of the right knee. Grasp the right ankle. Breathe well, and hold this pose for as long as is comfortable.

Release your leg, loosen up, and repeat the whole thing all over again on the other side.

In Sanskrit this position is called Ardha Matsyendrasana. As with all the spinal stretches and twists, it helps keep the spine mobile.

Shoulder variation of Ardha Matsyendrasana

Again, from a sitting-on-the-heels position, tilt to one side so that you can raise your right knee, slide your left heel under the raised right knee and place the heel close to your right buttock. Cross your right knee over your left leg, placing your right heel close to the left thigh.

Now raise your right arm over your head and place it with the palm open and on your back. Your elbow should be resting against the side of your head. Breathe, and try to move your palm down your back.

Now raise your left hand and reach behind you to try and touch the fingers of your other hand. This time, the elbow will be tucked in to the side of your body.

Add to this movement by twisting your upper body to the left, as if looking over your left shoulder. Hold the position before you exhale and twist to the other side, to the right.

6 Sit with the legs straight out in front of you, keeping your knees straight. If this is difficult to begin with think of tightening the front thigh muscles to achieve this straightness: you will very soon be elastic enough to flatten your knees without effort.

   Breathing out, bend forward from the spine and the hips (not the waist) and lean over your legs so that you can hold the soles of your feet with your hands.

As you become more supple you will find you can place your hands on the floor beyond your feet and rest your face close to your legs, but this takes time.

You will find that you do this in several 'goes': breathe well, and each time you breathe out you'll find that your body allows you a bit more reach.

Repeat several times.

At the very beginning, if you are very stiff, don't worry: place a belt or a dog lead round the soles of your feet and use this as a lever to help you bend forward and get closer to your feet.

Variation

Sit with your legs as wide apart as you can. To begin with this may not be very far. Breathe in, and raise your arms above your head, palms facing forwards.

Now slowly bend forward so that your palms and body are resting on the floor in front of you: your legs should remain as wide apart as they were at the beginning, but be careful not to let the knees roll inwards, they should be pointing up.

You may be disappointed with the fact that, at the beginning, you cannot get your legs very far apart while still bending your body forward to the floor. Don't worry: remember to breathe in and out, and that every new breath will help you to achieve more.

7 This is a simple spinal twist, the Sanskrit name of which is meru vakrasana.

Sit on the floor with your legs straight out in front of you. Raise either your left or right leg, bend it at the knee and place it over the leg that remains straight. If you have placed your left knee over your right leg, for example, bring your right arm round and cradle your left knee. Now place your left hand behind your back and turn your head round to the left: look up. Don't tense your neck or shoulders; try to keep them loose and your shoulders down: it's your spine that is working.

Bring your head back round and drop your chin on to your chest, as near as you can to your right shoulder. Breathe well. Bring your left shoulder forward, and then back. Now move your chin over to your left shoulder, which you pull backwards again. Repeat several times, then change over to the other side.

Standing poses

Standing poses in yoga make the legs and spine
supple and strong. Good posture and balance are
developed, thus increasing the sense of wellbeing and
personal power.

The standing forward bend (Pada hasthasana)

In essence, this pose involves bending over and
touching your toes. It looks so easy, and for the
young and the supple it is. The older we get,
however, and the more sedentary our lives, the
further we seem to get away from our toes!

If you did no other yoga exercise ever, a few
moments a day doing this will help to keep you
youthful. It lengthens the spine and helps to keep
that all-important part of the body flexible, as well as
easing the joints, stretches the hamstrings and legs
and increasing the supply of blood to the brain –
necessary for feeling clear-headed and vigorous.

Stand with your feet together and the weight of
your body on the balls of your feet. Check that your
shoulders are relaxed and your buttocks tucked in.
Raise your arms above your head, palms together, and
reach as high as you can. Feel the stretch from your
armpits to your hips.

Breathe out, bend forward from the hips and let
the crown of your head drop towards the floor. Catch
hold of your legs as far down as you can – if possible,

grasp your ankles lightly, but if not, hold your knees or calves.

Tuck your forehead in towards your legs and keep your knees straight but not rigidly locked. Check that your back is not rounded: your hips and buttocks should be pointing and stretching upwards.

Hold this position for as long as you find it comfortable, coming upright slowly to avoid feeling dizzy.

A variation on this is to place your arms as far round your legs as possible and to catch hold of the elbows with your hands. Some very supple folk are also able to bring the forefingers of each hand round their big toes, holding the toes slightly off the floor by these finger circles.

The Triangle (Trikonasana)

Stand upright, with the feet a little more than shoulder width apart. Spend a moment making sure your weight is distributed equally over both feet. Pull in your navel: this ensures that your bottom is tucked in. Breathe well, keeping your shoulders relaxed and your arms hanging loosely by your sides,

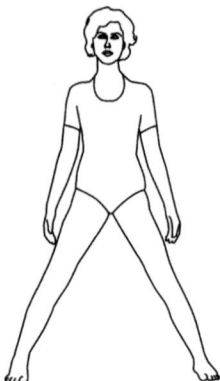

Breathe in, and bring your right arm straight up alongside your right ear. Feel the stretch in your rib cage and up the right side of your body.

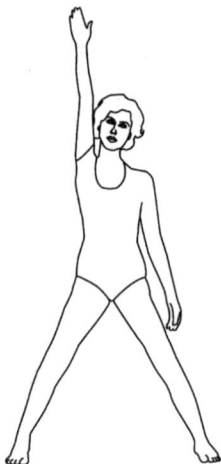

As you exhale, bend your body to the left, sliding your left hand as far down down your left leg as possible. After a while, you will easily manage to touch your left knee and perhaps soon the ankle. Hold the position for as long as is comfortable, remembering to breathe. As you breathe, you may find that each exhaled breath helps you to slide your left hand down a little more. Keep your right arm straight and level with your head and your right ear.

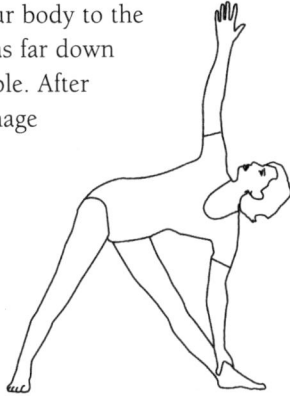

Don't bend your knees. When you have held this as long as comfortable, return to the upright position, breathe, and repeat with the left arm raised and your right hand sliding down your right leg.

Repeat again, both sides.

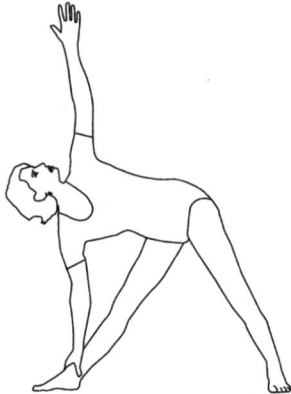

When you have finished, loosen up by shaking both legs and bending at the knees. Another useful 'loosener' is to shake the foot as if you are trying to detach it from your leg.

This one of the basic asanas or positions in yoga, and as with all the positions there are many variations on it.

Here are four that you can run on as a sequence after doing the basic Trikonasana.

I Stand in the basic position, then turn your right foot out so that it is pointing away from your body. The heel of your right foot should be in line with the centre of your left foot, which remains pointing forwards.

Raise your arms out to your sides and hold them at shoulder height.

Bend your right knee so that it is held over the right ankle, while keeping the left leg straight. Raise your left arm over your head and bend to the right.

It is important to try and keep your centre of gravity in your hips and trunk area, and not to lean too far forwards or backwards. Bring your right arm down and rest it on the bent right knee. Your left arm meanwhile will form a straight line that stretches up from the left ankle, the stretched and straight left leg, opening the rib cage and the side of the body and stretching up into the arm and fingertips.

Hold for as long as this is comfortable, then push your right arm off your knee and gradually come upright.

Loosen up by bending at the knees and shaking your legs.

As you become more supple, it is possible to vary this: instead of resting the un-stretched arm on the bent knee, place the hand of that arm flat on the floor alongside the foot of the knee that is bending. This will give you an even longer stretch with the other arm.

2 Stand with the feet slightly more than shoulder width apart, turn the right foot out so that the heels of your feet are at a 90 degree angle from each other. Lace your fingers together behind your back. Keep your left foot pointing straight ahead.

Breathe out and lunge forwards, trying to bring your forehead in contact with your right knee. At the same time your arms, with the fingers still laced, will come up straight behind you.

Arms and legs and knees should all be kept as straight as you can, but don't 'lock' them. The aim, when you are very supple, is to be able to rest your face against your right knee, but don't expect to do this straight away. In the meantime, keep breathing!

Breathe in as you come to the upright position

again, and repeat on the left side, turning your left foot out but keeping your right foot pointing straight ahead of you.

A variation on this, which helps the beginner, is to bend the knee of the foot that is turned out. Make sure the knee is over the foot: that is, when you look down you should see your knee and your toes, not your ankle or your foot. Clasp your hands behind your back and bend towards the bent knee, but this time, try to rest your forehead on the knee that is bending.

As always in these positions, gently return to the upright position, loosen your legs and feet, and repeat on the other side.

3   Stand in the basic triangle, feet apart but straight, and raise your arms at your sides to shoulder height. Look straight ahead, and ensure that you and 'centred' – that is, that you are neither leaning too far forwards or backwards, and your centre over gravity is in your solar plexus, weight distributed equally over both feet.

Moving from the hips (not the waist), try to bring your left hand to the ground outside your right foot. The right arm should be stretched up behind you, fingers pointing up. It may take a while to get to the floor – don't worry, rest your left hand on your right leg as far down as you can. Hold for a few moments before returning to the

upright position, and repeating with your right
hand and your left foot.

4   Stand upright, with your hands to nemaste. Now
bring your arms up to shoulder level, so that your
elbows are stretching out to either side and your
fingertips are touching in front of your breast-
bone. From the head down, you are making the
shape of a T.

Jump lightly to open your legs apart, opening
your arms at the same time. Now you are making
the shape of a star, with arms stretched out a
shoulder level, fingers together, and your legs are
under them. Don't have your legs to wide apart or
you will lose balance. Toes pointing forward.

Turn your right knee and foot to the right.
Bend your right knee, making a 90 degree angle
with the floor, but keep your spine straight. Your
abdomen and body should, however, remain
pointing forward and 'grounded'. To get out of this
pose, push off your right foot and return it to the
side of your left, so that you are once again
upright. Shake legs and arms to loosen up. Repeat
with the left knee.

This pose is known as **The Warrior**. The chest
and body are fully opened, the right arm and
thighs and calves all working – it induces a
wonderful feeling of inner power and strength,
without aggression.

The Tree

This pose is all about balance: it also tones and strengthens the legs. Any exercises that demand a certain degree of balance – and develop balance – are associated with heightening mental powers.

Stand upright, and check that you are balanced on both feet, with your body centred and your weight distributed evenly. Your arms should be hanging loosely by your sides. Breathe well and fix your eyes on a point straight in front of you. For many people this will just be a point on a blank wall, but if there is something at eye level to focus on – a picture, a real tree outside perhaps, a beam of light – so much the better.

Now shift your balance to the left foot and slide your right foot up your left leg as high as you can. Some people find it helps to guide the right foot into position with a hand.

The aim is to rest your right foot (or whichever foot it is you are bending) against the inner thigh of the leg which is supporting you. However, don't expect to do this in your first lesson! Many people start off by managing to rest the lifted foot against the ankle, calf or knee of the supporting leg – don't worry.

Once you are balanced, bring your hands to nemaste (the prayer position). Keeping the palms together, raise your hands high above your head, as tall as you can. Keep the crown of your head balanced over your body, and focus on the point straight ahead you have chosen. Feel the stretch upwards and remember the name of this pose: you are a tree, with your roots holding you firmly in the earth and nourishing you, and your beautiful, supple body reaching up to the brilliant sky.

Hold this position, breathing well, for as long as is comfortable and then slowly lower your arms to nemaste again, lower your foot, and loosen up both hands and legs.

When you have loosened up, repeat with the other foot.

The wobble factor inevitably affects newcomers to this pose. If you start to wobble or lose your balance, simply put your foot down, rest, focus your eyes in front of you and start again. Often it's possible to come out of a wobble simply by focusing your eyes and stretching upwards. Certain things cause wobbles: looking down, for instance, or bending your elbows, or bending the supporting knee, or not holding the bent leg on the inside of the supporting leg.

Remember that once you were a small child and needed stabilisers or a firm parental hand to help you stay on a bicycle at all. And then one day, after many wobbles, you just woke up able to balance on that extraordinary machine, and never looked back! It will be the same with yoga.

Natarajasana: the Cosmic Dancer

This asana takes its name from an incarnation of the god Shiva as Nataraja, 'the king of the dancers': destroying and recreating the Universe in a ever-repeating cycle of death and renewal. This is an asana that develops balance, so it makes sense to practice this in a sequence after The Tree.

Stand upright, focusing your eyes on a point straight ahead of you. Spend a moment checking that you are centred and balanced. Breathe well.

Raise your left leg behind you so that you can reach back and hold the foot, bringing it close to your left buttock. Keep your right leg straight but relaxed. Don't tense your shoulders.

Breathe in, and stretch your right arm above your head, palm facing forwards. Check that you are focusing on a point ahead of you at eye level. Keep your chin level: neither down on your chest, nor pulling your head back.

Keeping your right arm upright and straight, push your left leg away from your body as if you were trying to straighten it, and bend forwards. As you bend forwards, you will have to bring your head down and shift your focus to a point on the floor. Keep your raised arm straight, close to your ear.

Looked at in outline, the front half of the body looks like a swimmer, diving into clear cool water: but the left arm is still holding on to the left ankle, which is pushing away from the body, trying to be parallel to the ground.

Imagine that the body parts at either end of you – the raised right arm and the clasped left foot – are trying to stretch you taller, reaching away from each other.

The balance is difficult, so keep breathing. Hold for as long as you can. Repeat with the other foot and the other arm raised.

The Dog (Swanasana)

As stated earlier, many yoga positions take their names from the animal kingdom. There are many reasons for this, one being the observation that animals are so comfortable and integrated within their own bodies; humans, sadly, seldom are. It is a good aim in life to observe the grace and beauty of animal movements (as dancers have over the centuries) and try to emulate their fluidity and flexibility.

One thing animals do, for health, is stretch. Instinctively, they exercise their muscles by stretching them, holding and releasing – a pattern we know is vital for health and suppleness.

Begin the dog pose by sitting on your knees. If this is not comfortable for you, remember to push a cushion between your heels and your buttocks. Sit upright, and then crouch forward. Rest your forehead on the floor in front of you, and your hands, palms facing down, resting on the floor just above your head. Rest your forearms on the floor.

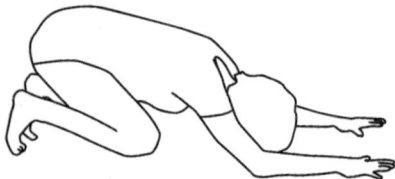

Tuck your toes under your feet, lift your head and push yourself up by your elbows – your elbows will straighten and your feet can now take the weight of your body. Keep your elbows straight and push your buttocks up. Try to put your heels on the floor: if you keep your elbows and legs straight you may not be able to do this, and will feel a real 'pull' on the backs of your legs.

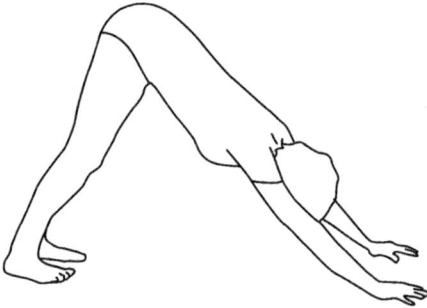

Spend a moment checking your arms and elbows are straight, your buttocks are up, your back is straight, and that you are keeping your legs straight too – try to inch your heels so that they are flat on the floor and your body is forming an inverted v shape, but don't worry if you can't: this is really hard work on the hamstrings and takes practice. Feel the pull on the backs of your legs but don't over-do it.

Hold the position, then lower your knees to the floor and relax by adopting the Pose of the Child (see facing page) – although if you are coming out of the Dog, you should miss out the first stage and just lie with your forehead on the floor in the second stage of that pose.

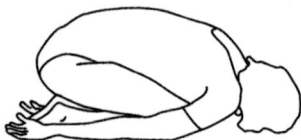

The Pose of the Child

This is a comforting pose and recommended when you come out of any sequence of poses such as the Dog or the Cat that stretches you in every sense of the word. If you are very stressed or tired or unhappy, take up this pose for a few moments, breathing well, comforting yourself in the way you might comfort and reassure a child.

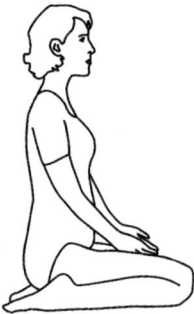

Sit back on your knees: if this is not comfortable for you, place a cushion or a foam pad between your heels and your buttocks.

Breathe out and bend forward slowly until your forehead is resting on the floor in front of you. Your feet should still be side by side, but release any tension or 'hold' in them. Your arms should be lying loosely by your side, against your body and on the floor, with the palms facing upwards. If your neck or shoulders feel tense, focus on releasing them by breathing well.

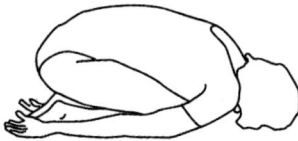

If you can hold this position for a few moments, while breathing easily, you can use it to repeat a mantra, or a calming affirmation, or for a visualisation. See Chapter 4 for examples of these.

The Cat

Cats have an enviable physical grace: their movements seem unhurried, purposeful, fluid. Although cats never 'exercise' in the sense of running around in the way, for instance, that a dog does, stretching forms a major part of their daily ritual. This pose emulates that stretching routine, and is wonderful for relieving tension and stress. If you are prone to back pain through stress, try to do this every day.

Sit back on your knees, with your heels tucked under you, as you were for the Pose of the Child. Lean forward and place your forearms and hands on the ground in front of you.

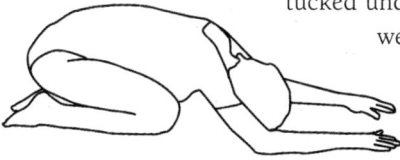

Now raise your body from the hips, keeping your knees and hands on the floor, so that you make the shape of a table. Your hands and arms and knees should be supporting you equally so they need to be under your body. Your back, which is the table top, should be flat. Take care not to round it.

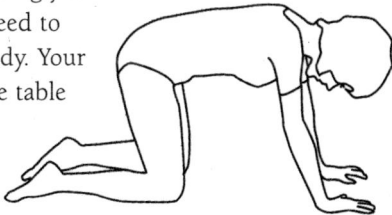

133

Breathe in, and arch your back: as you breathe out, drop your head forward so that it is resting between your arms. Try to visualise that it is your back that is arching, not your shoulders. Keeping your head down will help also to keep your shoulders down too.

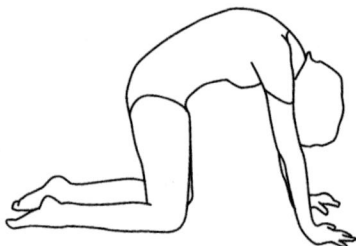

Inhale again, lower your chest, bend your elbows and raise your chin As you do so, your back will become concave– imagine a hollow in the middle of your back that you could pour milk into!

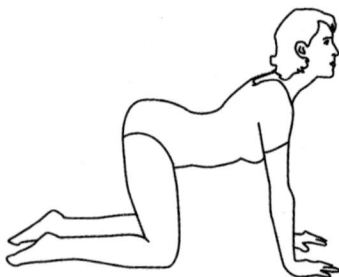

Repeat the stage described above, of arching your back: arms straight, head down.

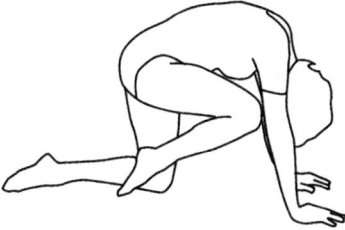

Now return to the 'table' position you held first. Breathe in, and pull your left knee under you as if you are trying to touch your chest with it. Hold, and then stretch your left leg out behind you, pointing your toe straight out. Raise your chin, look upwards, and make sure your elbows and relaxed: bend them a little if you wish to give you support as you focus on really stretching your leg out behind you.

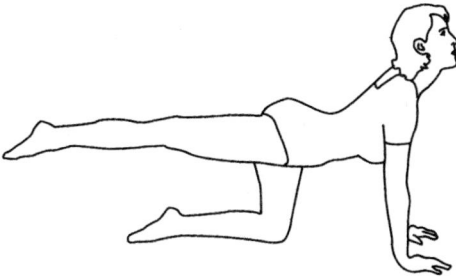

Once again, pull your left knee under your chest and then rest it on the floor. Check your breathing.

Now repeat with the right leg.

135

The Cobra

This asana is recommended for women suffering from PMT or menstrual disorders, and for those who suffer from digestive problems.

From a kneeling or sitting position, lower yourself face down on the floor. Your legs should be together, but not tightly so, and your feet lying relaxed. Don't tuck your toes under. Relax for a few moments with your head to one side so that you are resting on a cheek, and tuck your arms under your head. Breathe and close your eyes.

To come in to the Cobra, place your hands level with your chest and your forehead on the floor. Make sure that it is your forehead you are resting on the floor, or your neck may be strained. Check also that your palms are level with your chest and not higher.

Keeping your legs together, raise your elbows off the floor, preparing to support your upper body.

Breathe in, raise your forehead off the floor, and look up so that your chin follows.

Now try to point your chin at the ceiling, so that your head is held back and your chest rises. Lift your chest off the floor as high as you can, and use your palms to give yourself more leverage.

Keep your tummy on the floor and your shoulders down and relaxed – your chest and arms are doing the work. Don't straighten your arms. Don't confuse the Cobra with the press-ups that sports people do: the purpose of press-ups is to work the biceps of the arms, but in the Cobra the purpose is to feel stretch along the spine. It's as if you are rolling your body up from the head end, lengthening and extending your spine.

Hold the position for as long as is comfortable and then slowly fold yourself back down again, starting with the spine: imagine that you are placing one vertebra after another flat on the floor until your body is once again entirely in contact with the floor, then lower your head last of all.

Turn your head to one side and place it on your folded arms to relax.

Variations

There are several variations on the basic cobra pose. In all of them, though, it is important to keep your abdomen flat on the floor.

In Variation 1, raise your palms off the floor and keep your elbows back. Your body is arching up as much as possible, and as you roll upwards into the Cobra position you are making your back muscles work really hard.

In Variation 2, clasp your hands – with fingers laced – over your buttocks before you rise up from the head. When you are as high as you can get, push your hands away from you, keeping your arms straight. Hold for as long as is comfortable.

In Variation 3, do Variation 2 but then push your palms towards the ceiling, raising your arms as high as you can. This is good for increasing suppleness in your shoulders and upper back.

King Cobra is an advanced pose that even quite supple people can find difficult. It should not be attempted by pregnant women or those with a history of back pain. To achieve this, you need to lie face down with your legs slightly apart. As you rise up with the head and chest, use your hands to "walk" your body backwards. Bend the knees and bring the feet to meet your head as it curls back. Your tummy will have to lift off the floor but you must keep your hips and buttocks firmly down. Your palms remain on the floor in front of you.

The Locust

This asana counter-poses the Cobra, and is excellent both for those with digestive problems and women who wish to tone and strengthen the pelvic floor area.

Lie on your stomach, chin on the floor, legs straight. Keeping your arms straight by your sides, clench your fists and bring them together in the area of your groin. The point of this asana is to keep your fists clenched while you raise both legs together behind you.

The legs are immensely heavy objects to lift, even in the lightest people, so it is recommended that you begin with what is called a half-Locust. That is, follow the instructions as above, but instead of raising both legs, breathe in deeply and raise one leg off the floor, keeping it straight and raising it as high as you can. Raise your hip as well as your leg. Hold for as long as is comfortable, then lower the leg, breathe well, and repeat with the other leg.

Once you have had some practice in this, try the full Locust, raising both legs, hips and bottom off the floor, and holding for as long as is comfortable.

The Fish

Lie flat on the floor with your legs and feet together; do not bend your knees. Slide your hands under your buttocks, so that you are lying on the backs of your hands; if you do not wish to do this you can keep your arms lying by your side, but keep the palms and the elbows on the floor. Using your elbows to push you, raise your chest up in an arch and move your head back until the crown of your head is resting on the floor behind you. Make sure it is the crown of your head and not just the back of your head.

Your shoulders should be off the floor, and the body is being supported by your elbows. This is why it is best if you can rest your hands on your buttocks, as this ensures that your elbows are under your body, taking its weight. There will be an arch under your neck, with the shoulders on one side and the back of the head on the other. Keep your feet together, legs straight and buttocks on the floor. As always, breathe well.

To come out of this pose, lift your head slightly, and gently lower your shoulders and back down to the floor.

This pose has the Sanskrit name of Matsyasana. In yoga classes or in sequences of poses it is often used as the counter-balance to the shoulder stand (see below), and after the Fish many people go into the Corpse (also below).

Variation

Sit cross-legged on the floor, knees raised off the
floor, holding on to your feet, and then slowly lie on
your back, keeping your legs crossed beneath you.
Carry on holding your feet, so that when you lie
down your hands will be straight by your side,
reaching down to your feet.

Now use your elbows to push you off the floor,
arching the chest as before and maintaining your
weight on your elbows. Rest the crown of your head
on the floor, releasing any tension you can feel in
your neck or shoulders. Breathe deeply and easily.
Keep your knees on the floor.

When you wish to come out of this position,
gently lower your head and neck to the floor. Raise
your arms above your head and rest them on the
floor, holding your elbows above your head. Breathe
deeply.

Yoga mudra

This pose is often used in conjunction with the variation on the Fish described above. Sit cross-legged and lean forward until your forehead is resting on the floor in front of you. If you cannot reach the floor comfortably, use a cushion or a foam pad for your forehead. Reach your hands behind you and lock fingers at the level of your hips. Breathe well.

Breathe in and, as you breathe out, raise your clasped hands vertically behind you, keeping them as straight as possible. Hold this pose for as long as is comfortable. On an out breath, straighten up and release your hands to your sides.

Roll your shoulders to loosen them up after this pose.

The Shoulder stand

Raising the feet and legs above the head is an important part of yoga practice, and brings great health benefits. It has a resting, invigorating effect on the whole body, relieving stress and making natural sleep possible.

If you don't want to do a shoulder stand However, please don't be put off – and miss out on the benefits – by the thought of doing difficult or complicated poses that seem to demand a certain level of athletic skill.

If you can't or don't wish to do any kind of shoulder stand, simply find a wall or a door (uncluttered by radiators or handles) and rest your feet against them for several minutes. Get into position by lying on the floor with knees bent and your feet as close as you can get them to the wall or door. Lift your legs and shuffle your bottom forwards, again so that you are as close as possible to the wall. You are aiming to lie in the shape of a capital L.

Rest your arms loosely by your side, close your eyes and rest like this. The effect is calming and you may wish to choose this time to do a visualisation, or simply reflect on your life and the issues of concern to you.

To come out of this, bend your knees and roll over on to your side.

To do a shoulder stand, start by lying flat on your back; raise your legs in the air and bend your knees and, as you push your legs up off the floor, place both hands in the small of your back and use them to push yourself. Keep your elbows flat on the floor. Don't rush this, or you will wobble and fall over. Slowly and gently, straighten your legs in the air and hold that position, supported by your elbows on the floor and your hands firmly supporting your back.

To come down, lower your legs gently, supporting your back all the while. Again, don't come down too quickly and risk hurting your back.

This is the basic shoulder stand and there are many variations – some quite demanding – upon this position. One is to move into the Plough, which is described below.

The Plough

Begin the Plough from the
basic Shoulder stand. Your
chin is resting against your
neck, the back and legs are
as straight as possible, feet
together, elbows and
shoulders close to the body
which is being supported
by the hands. Be conscious
of your breathing.

As you breathe out,
gently lower your legs so
that your toes touch the
floor behind your head.
Beginners may not be able
to touch the floor; that will

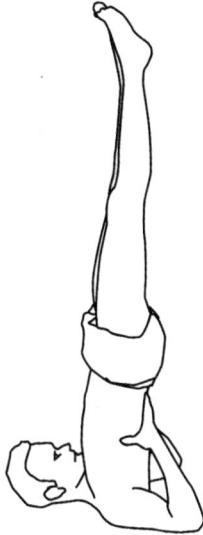

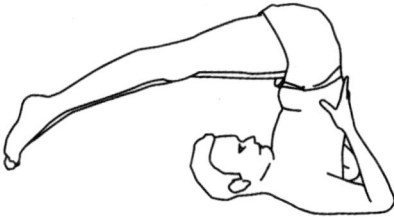

come. For the moment, lower your legs as far as
possible behind your head without losing your
balance. Keep the legs straight and the feet together,
for once you lose that your balance may go too.

If you can, tuck your toes under and rest them on the floor behind your head keeping the legs straight. The way to do this is to ensure that your back is also upright and your hips are 'pushing' towards the ceiling.

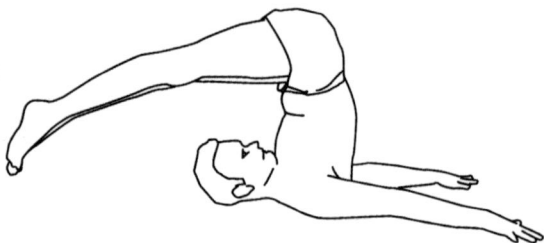

Now slide your arms out flat, so that the palms are resting on the floor, away from your feet. You are now precisely in the shape of a traditional wooden Plough.

To come out of this position, resume the Shoulder stand and gently lower yourself to the floor, supporting your back with your hands as you do so.

The Corpse

In spite of its somewhat grim name, this simple pose is truly relaxing. (Its Sanskrit name, Sarvasana, sounds much more peaceful.) You should adopt this after any strenuous pose and many yoga classes end with a few moments in this pose for the purposes of relaxation. Use it at home if you are particularly tired or stressed, or need a period in which to think and reflect calmly. One thing, though: the body temperature falls dramatically when you lie like this, so if you are not in a warm room, cover yourself with a blanket or put on extra clothing. In a yoga class, this is the moment to put your socks and a sweatshirt back on.

All you have to do is lie flat on the floor with your legs apart and your arms away from the body, the hands and fingers falling naturally open. Consider in turn each body part from your toes upwards and make a conscious effort to relax it, releasing tension. Pay attention to your breathing but don't 'do' breathing: just be.

The Rabbit
Kneel up on the floor, toes tucked under, so that your bottom is resting on your upraised heels. Breathe in, and as you breathe out, bend forward and place your forehead as close as you can to your knees.

Now roll on to your crown. Raise your hips in the air and straighten your elbows. Your back should not be hunched, though it will be rounded. Try to keep your shoulders relaxed. Hold for as long as is comfortable, return to your original position, and then repeat.

Any asana that involves a fresh supply of oxygenated blood to the brain is both calming and invigorating.

The Crocodile

Lie on your abdomen with your head tucked inward and down and your forehead resting on top of your folded fore arms. The legs should be a comfortable distance apart, with your feet and toes pointing outward. Always breathe fully, feeling the abdomen expanding downward with each inhalation and your hips and buttocks rising slightly upward with the exhalation. Allow the gentle movement to soothe your pre menstrual cramping and massage the uterine muscles.

The child's pose

As previously, you should kneel with your buttocks
resting on your heels. Bend at the hips and let your
torso relax on your thighs and your forehead rest on
the floor. Relax your arms and hands on the floor
beside you with the palms up and the fingers
pointing toward your feet. Place a pillow either on
your lap if you are having difficulty folding your body
over your thighs, or between your calves and thighs if
you cannot rest comfortably on your heels.

The Camel

This is a good exercise not only for stretching the whole spine, but also for opening the chest.

Kneel upright, with back straight, hands loosely at your side. Check that your hips are above your knees, so that you are neither leaning backwards nor forwards. Slip your arms behind your back at level with your lower back (just above your buttocks) and grasp your elbows.

Breathe in, push your hips forward and lean your head back, keeping your face up. Breathe well.

Chin still pointing upwards, take your hands back until they are touching your heels. Your hips are forward. Check that your neck and facial muscles are relaxed. Hold for as long as is comfortable.

To rest from this position, come forward and rest your forehead on the ground in front of you. You can then come into the Pose of the Child.

The Bridge

This is a simple asana but, as with so many asanas, it has some very advanced and challenging variations. It strengthens the wrists and arms, but is also reported as beneficial in easing period pains and strengthening the pelvic floor after childbirth.

Lie flat on the floor with your arms at your sides. Bring your knees up so that your feet are lying close to your buttocks. Feet and knees are slightly apart but level. They should not be further apart than your body width.

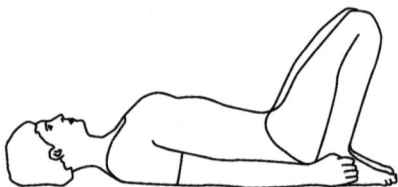

Now raise your hips high off the ground, and support your lower back with your hands, fingers inwards and thumb round your waist. The hips and chest are lifting as high as possible (making, of course, the shape of a bridge) but your feet remain firmly on the floor, as do head, neck and shoulders. Your elbows are flat on the floor, supporting the arms. Hold for as long as is comfortable: when you lower your body, take care not to jar your neck.

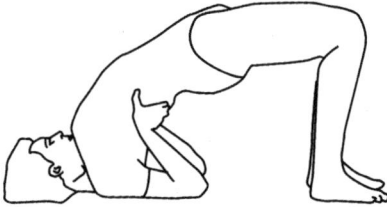

When you come out of a pose such as this, it is good to remain flat on the floor and bring your knees up to your chest, cradling them in your arms. Roll around clockwise and anti-clockwise on the floor, ensuring that your spine touches the floor.

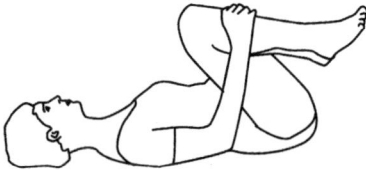

Variation 1

Adopt the Bridge position and, when you are there, raise one leg in the air above your body. Point with the toe. At the same time, be careful that your hips do not 'collapse' – it should feel as if your raised leg is pulling your hips up with them, while your other leg remains stable. Lower the leg gently, and then repeat with the other one, breathing well as you do so.

To come out of this pose, retain the bridge with your hips raised off the floor, chest raised, both legs on the floor, and place your hands on the top of your thighs. Gradually lower yourself to the floor.

As with any exercise where you have placed weight on your head and neck, loosen up by rolling your head from side to side with your eyes closed.

Variation 2

This should not be attempted until you have been practising for a few months and are quite at ease with the Shoulder stand. To begin this variation on the Bridge, adopt the Shoulder stand, so that your legs are straight up in the air above your body, your elbows forming a 'bracket' on the ground and your hands firmly supporting your back.

Slowly bend your knees and drop first one knee, then the other. If you drop both knees together you may lose your balance. One after the after, drop your feet to the ground, keeping your hips high. Don't raise your head. Now hold the Bridge for as long as is comfortable, breathing well, and then either return to the Shoulder stand (lifting one leg, then the other) or sink gently the floor.

The Sun Salutation

This is a complete sequence made up of twelve
individual poses, each of which balances the other. If
you can practice this daily, or whenever you do your
yoga, you will develop flexibility and suppleness: and
it is an excellent warm-up for other asanas.

When you are familiar with it, you should aim to
perform the Sun Salutation as one unbroken
sequence. A complete sequence requires that the
movements are repeated twice, as you will lead with
one leg first, and then need to repeat with the other.
It does not matter whether you begin with the left or
the right foot as long as you repeat with the other. Of
course, you can repeat the entire cycle as often as you
wish, but try to do it at least twice to start with,
gradually building up.

Try not to move your hands between positions 3
and 6. Don't forget to breathe in rhythm with your
movements, and don't strain. If at any time you feel
tension in your neck or shoulders or back, try to
release that tension by slowing down and breathing
more deeply.

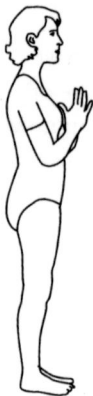

1 Stand upright with your hands at nemaste, the prayer position. Your thumbs should be resting against your breast bone. Your feet should be together.

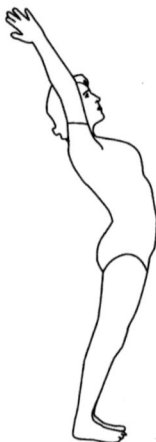

2 Breathe in, raise your arms above your head and, from the waist, arch backwards as far as is comfortable: your hips will be pushed forward. Keep your legs straight.

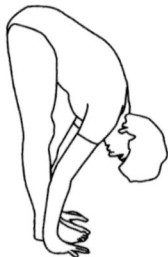

3 Breathe out, and bend forward from the hips, reaching down to your feet. Drop your head. Place your hands, palms down, beside your feet: toes and fingers should be level. You may need to bend your knees

to do this, but don't worry about that – what's important is that your hands and feet are level for the next stage.

4 Whether you are 'doing' the left or the right leg this time – and for the sake of this description we'll start with the left – slide that leg out behind you and rest the knee on the floor, with the toes tucked under. You will be crouching on your right knee, rather like a runner waiting for the starting gun.

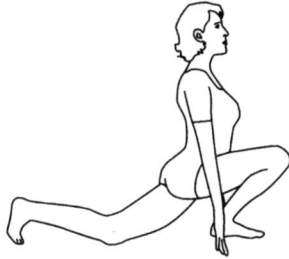

5 Slide the other leg out behind you, again with toes tucked under, so that now you are raised on both hands, which are supporting you, with both legs out behind you, raised on the toes. Hold this position.

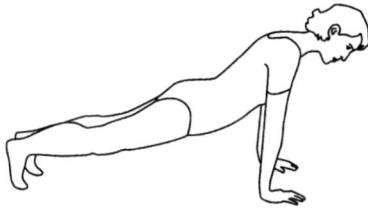

157

6 Breathing out, lower your knees, chest and touch the floor with your forehead. Keep your toes tucked under you, and your hips slightly raised.

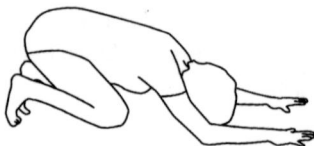

7 Take a deep breath, uncurl your toes and point them straight out behind you; now raise yourself again on your arms, which are close to your body and level with your shoulders, and raise your chin, tilting your head back. Your hips should be on the floor, shoulders down and back, and elbows slightly bent as your hands push you up away from the floor.

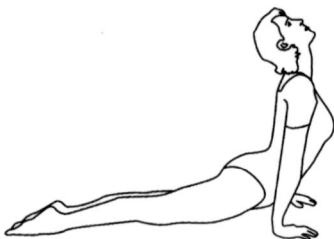

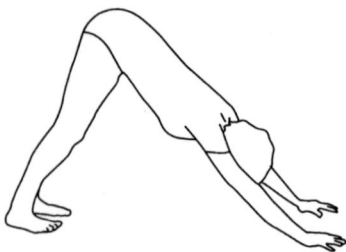

8 Tuck your toes under your feet so that you can push yourself up into the Dog pose. Remember that in the Dog you are

trying to make the shape of an inverted v: supported on your hands, which are flat on the ground, head dropped between your arms, feet flat on the floor.

9 From this, drop into the same position as in 4 but with the other leg. That is, this time slide the right leg out behind you, toes tucked under, and crouch on the left knee which is bent between your hands. Hold and stretch for a moment.

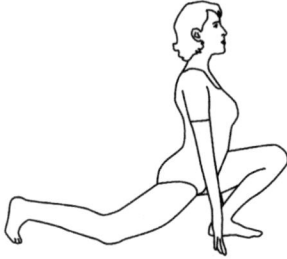

10 Then, as in 3, bring your right leg forward and raise yourself upright on both legs to the standing position. Your hands, however, should remain level with your feet, so you may need to bend your knees to achieve this.

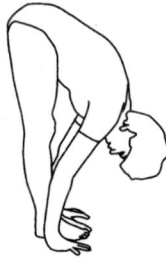

11 Raise yourself slightly from the floor and bring your hands to nemaste. As you do so, breathe in and raise your arms above your ahead and then arch yourself backwards again, bending over slowly and deliberately and not forcing the movement.

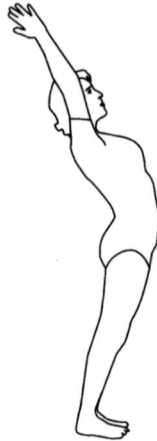

12 Breathe out, come gently back to the upright position, and drop your hands loosely by your side. You have completed the Sun Salutation.

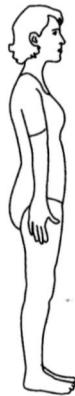

As its name implies, the Sun Salutation has its origins in ancient Hindu practice in homage to the sun, celebrated, as in other religions, as a powerful symbol of life, warmth, health and immortality. Traditionally these asanas are performed at sunrise as a welcome to the dawning day.

CHAPTER 4
Yoga and Health Benefits

The practice of yoga is very beneficial in many ways. It is good not only for the prevention of disease, but it also has many therapeutic properties, which can help to improve certain health problems. Two such problems that can be helped and greatly improved are asthma and arthritis.

When you go to a yoga therapist for help with a particular condition or simply for one-to-one yoga training, the first step is usually an assessment of your condition and overall situation. This involves going for an individual session (60–90 minutes) with a qualified yoga therapist. To save time you would usually complete a questionnaire in advance and post it in. You will then be directed to a class, course or further one-to-one sessions as best suits your individual needs. Should a one-to-one session not be necessary, you will usually be advised on the best class or course. All specialist classes are taught by yoga therapists. These are yoga teachers with a further two years of medically based training.

What is yoga therapy?

Yoga is the adaptation of yoga for people with health problems. Although general yoga classes can improve general health and resolve mild complaints, they may be ineffective – or even harmful – for serious conditions. In such cases, yoga therapy can help people by tailoring yoga to their individual needs, taking into account their health problems, constitution and circumstances. Yoga therapy uses the traditional practises from India, which date back thousands of years and were part of their traditional health care system. These practices are among the most effective known methods for managing stress-related conditions, which are so common today. This is because they bridge the gap between body and mind.

Yoga is a dynamic system of physical exercise and a valuable philosophy to apply to everyday life. The ultimate goal of yoga philosophy is complete detachment from reality, as we understand it, and complete self knowledge or Samadhi. Only by separating yourself from the environment can you come to terms with your individual personality and start putting the mind and emotions in complete order. This lack of self knowledge is thought to be the fundamental cause of many emotional and nervous problems. Yoga aims to deal with that and put it to right.

Far too often yoga is practised purely as a physical exercise or to improve ones concentration or ease tension. Whilst it may well be useful for all these purposes, to be successful in yoga the ultimate goal of self realisation must always be the main aim as by working towards this aim we shall be assured of improved concentration, lack of tension etc. However if we are only interested in the side benefits of yoga it is unlikely we shall ever achieve what we set out to do.

The lack of natural exercise in our lives has left many people with chronic health and stress problems, especially as they get older. Yoga enables the student to find relief from these physical ailments and to strengthen the body and make it more supple.

Regular asana and pranayama practice will bring serenity and calmness to the student, enabling the internal organs to become strong and to work efficiently. By so doing the student can overcome many symptoms of stress, such as headaches, stiff necks, lower backache, insomnia and digestive disorders. Yoga practice helps to improve concentration and self-discipline, and to harness one's energy – by so doing, it brings vitality in your everyday activities.

From the psychological viewpoint, yoga sharpens the intellect and aids concentration. It steadies the emotions and encourages a caring concern for others. Above all, it gives hope. The practice of breathing techniques calms the mind. Its philosophy sets life in perspective. In the realm of the spiritual, yoga brings awareness and the ability to be still. Through meditation, inner peace is experienced. Thus yoga is a practical philosophy involving every aspect of a person's being. It teaches the evolution of the individual by the development of self-discipline and self-awareness. Anyone, irrespective of age, health, circumstance of life and religion, can practise yoga.

Interest in alternative or complementary therapies has increased noticeably in recent years, and a growing number of people daily seek professional help from practitioners of aromatherapy, acupuncture, homeopathy, reflexology and herbal medicine, to name but a few. Yoga belongs very firmly within that structure, not because it offers specific remedies for particular ailments – it is not a medical treatment – but because it belongs in a tradition both of holistic and preventative medicine.

The holistic tradition believes that mind and body are one, and that in treating an ailment the whole person must be treated, rather than just the ailment. Conventional Western medicine has tended to regard a disease or condition as if it was somehow separate from the human being that has it. A person suffering from, say, a digestive disorder, will be given medication or, drastically, surgery that is concerned only with suppressing the symptoms and removing the malignancy of that condition. A holistic practitioner starts from who the person is, asking for a detailed history of their lifestyle, state of mind and daily habits, believing that the origins of the disease or condition will be found there. Take for example the case of someone in a highly stressful job leading a high-octane life – travel, long hours of work, pressure at work, rushed meals of fast food, alcohol for stimulation and 'relaxation', perhaps cigarettes as well – who develops an ulcer. Conventional medicine would prescribe drugs to treat the ulcer; holistic medicine would recommend a change of lifestyle and re-ordered priorities – good food, good rest, a minimum of alcoholic stimulation, a more tranquil approach – in order not only to cure the ulcer but to prevent its recurrence; it's not just the disease that needs healing, but the person who has the ailment.

At the heart of the philosophy of yoga is a belief in balance. Not just the balance of the body – achieving poise and grace through controlled postures – but the balance of the mind, too. Many Eastern religions and philosophies have at their core a belief in the existence of opposites in a cycle of conflict with each other: yin and yang, light and dark, heat and cold, death and birth, good and bad. The tension between opposites is necessary for life, is indeed the essence of life: but the balance between the two must be maintained in harmony. Chaos and disorder follow when the balance is lost.

In our own lives, too, we know that a certain

amount of stress or tension is both unavoidable and necessary. The right amount of 'stress' – wanting to achieve, to do well, to pass an exam, to learn a new skill – drives us forward in a positive, challenging way. It is only when that stress becomes too much or is unreasonable or negative in origin (wanting to earn more money than other people, competing in an unhealthy way, working overly hard in a critical or negative environment) that our mental and physical health begins to deteriorate.

The practice of yoga teaches us that mind and body are one, and that when the body is relaxed and strong and supple so will the mind be also. It is impossible to practice yoga while feeling angry, tense or distressed. You might bring these emotions to a session, but once you start to breathe deeply and focus on the asanas such negativity dissolves and the mind is released from the prison of these feelings.

The following can be used and practised to benefit health problems.

- *Physical exercises*: Simple movements and held postures gently stretch and strengthen muscles, improve mobility, flexibility, respiration, circulation, digestion and elimination, and promote a general sense of health and well being.

- *Breathing techniques*: By controlling patterns of breathing, yoga can calm and centre the mind, helping to relieve stress and mental fatigue.

- *Relaxation*: A central element in yoga therapy, relaxation is the body's way of recharging and helps to ease physical and mental tensions.

- *Lifestyle*: By encouraging us to step back and look objectively at our habitual patterns of behaviour, yoga can help us to cope better with situations that put our bodies and minds under strain.

Will yoga therapy work for you?

If your problem is more serious than having a headache or menstruating, or if you are pregnant, you must inform your GP before starting any classes. This is for your own safety. Regular classes are not suitable for those with certain medical conditions. Please inform your doctor and your teacher *before* starting classes if you have any of the following conditions: heart disease or any heart problem, epilepsy including petit mal, cancer or benign tumours, diabetes, meniere's disease, detached retina, AIDS, MS (multiple sclerosis) or if you have recently had an operation.

Yoga therapy can help a wide range of medical conditions including arthritis, asthma and other respiratory disorders, cancer, diabetes, depression, high blood pressure, HIV and AIDS, low back pain, mental illness, ME, MS and women's health problems. It is also excellent for pregnancy, childbirth and babies and their mothers. Yoga therapy starts with very simple exercises. People can begin to practice and benefit right away, even if they have never done yoga before. Commencing with stretching and breathing exercises, students gradually progress in stages to a range of asanas, pranayama and relaxation practices. Yoga therapy retains the basic principles and aims of yoga, working holistically at all levels of the mind and body. Although clients may go for help with the specific intention of solving their health problems, they will benefit in many other ways. In fact, yoga therapy will be less effective if a holistic approach is not taken.

Stress is one of the mental problems where yoga can be helpful. We all need a certain amount of stress in our lives to give us motivation and encouragement to continue, but when it restricts our daily life to a great extent, it can become a major problem and will begin to affect our health. We are all very different individuals and what may be regarded as a positive stress for one person might have a very negative effect on another. It is important, therefore, that we can learn to recognise our own capabilities and find some ways of managing any of the stressful events in our lives. It is not always possible or practical to avoid some of the situations that can cause the stress, so we have to find an effective way of assisting our selves to cope with the situation. It is important that we should all learn to take responsibility for our own health and bodies, and Yoga is one way of achieving this – the vast numbers of people who now practice the art of yoga means that something must be working for them! Yoga asanas are particularly helpful in relation to stress as they have a profound effect on our whole mind and body. Our central nervous system is nourished by the spine, and the condition of our spine is largely responsible for our physical and emotional well being. In Yoga practice, the spine is the most exercised part of the body so it is easy to see what the benefits of Yoga practice may be. Yoga postures also help to stimulate the lymphatic system that will help to remove toxins from the body that, if allowed to accumulate, will no doubt cause much pain and stiffness in the muscles and joints. The functioning of the glands is also regulated, which will create the correct balance in our system.

As well as all of the postures in yoga, correct breathing is another important feature of yoga practice. Breathing is one of the most important functions of the body and all other functions depend on it. Most of us use only a fraction of our lung capacity, which actually results in tension in the neck and back, improper functioning of the digestive system and also a build up of toxins in the system. Benefits that can be gained from correct breathing are improved circulation, reduced tension, increased oxygen supply to all body cells and extra vitality due to more efficient supply of prana or life force throughout the body.

Lack of sleep

One of the major problems of today's stressful
lifestyles and jobs is that of stress, depression, and
more commonly insomnia, or lack of sleep. Insomnia
can happen even if you are feeling very sleepy or
physically tired. Often, the situation arises where you
desperately need to sleep so that you will be properly
rested and alert for going to work, or for a big night
out, but you simply end up staring wide eyed at the
bedroom ceiling. It can happen to anyone, even those
who are usually heavy sleepers and have never had
problems with sleep in the past. The symptoms are
that your mind is overactive and agitated, and your
body won't relax no matter how hard you try to relax
and sleep. The harder you work at getting to sleep,
the wider awake you end up becoming. Even if you
try all of the traditional methods of getting to sleep,
such as counting sheep, having a hot milky drink,
having a quick snack, having some light exercise, they
will generally be of very little success.

The problem of insomnia and stress is one of the
major causes of sleeping pills being prescribed in the
United States, where approximately one third of all
adults suffer from some type of sleep disorder.
Insomnia, the most common type by far, is clinically
defined as the inability to fall asleep after lying in bed
for thirty minutes, or the inability to sustain sleep for
more than a few hours without waking. Practically

speaking, however, insomnia can be defined as unrestful sleep, as the clinical description is actually very common now.

We have probably all experienced some form of insomnia at particularly stressful times in our lives. It is very normal to have trouble sleeping at these times, but the difference is that it usually passes after a night or two. Insomnia only becomes a major problem when it becomes chronic. Although the problem is associated with certain physical illnesses, such as arthritis, heart failure, and chronic lung disease, most experts agree that insomnia is a symptom of a problem and not an illness in itself. If you are wondering what it is a symptom of, I have actually mentioned the problem – life!

An ancient view of the problem...

Ayurveda, which is the healing science associated with yoga, tells us that each and every disease we will experience or suffer from is caused by indigestion. That is, at some level – either physical, mental, or emotional – we haven't completed the process of extracting what is helpful to us and eliminating what is indigestible. This is one of the keys to understanding insomnia.

On the physical level, indigestion can be caused either by bad food or by weak digestion and always leads to conditions like heartburn (which is a major contributor to the symptom of insomnia), flatulence, and diarrhoea. Similarly, we can compare this to the condition of mental indigestion, which is the inability to let go of a certain incident or thought – usually an unpleasant experience. This could be something distant from you, such as a plane crash that has been particularly tragic or any event where something upsetting to you has happened. This in turn will cause you to become upset to an extent, and you may think of it to an excess. It could also come from something that is directly related to you, such as criticism from someone whose opinion we value, or a work-related problem that you are trying to solve. Emotional indigestion is the repeat of a feeling, often sadness or anger, long after the event actually happened. The emotion has not been sufficiently digested and remains just under the surface, springing up for no apparent reason. An example of this would be the death of a family member years ago. Mental and emotional indigestion are always the most common causes of insomnia. Some of us even grind our teeth while we sleep in an attempt to chew and digest recurring thoughts and emotions.

The modern view...
Modern explanations for insomnia range from over-stimulation and stress to mucking up our waking-sleeping cycle, such as having a lie in at the weekends. Stimulants which we over-indulge in include caffeine (found in coffee, tea, chocolate, and

some fizzy drinks), and sugar, as well as activities such as aerobic exercise, arguing, and watching violent or exciting TV programmes. As with the ancient view, this would actually include watching or listening to news reports. All of these factors, if they are taken (or experienced) too close to bedtime, can tense us up so much that it is difficult to fall asleep. This is only another way of saying we are still attempting to digest these substances or events at the same time we are courting sleep. One of the major contributors to younger people having trouble sleeping is playing computer games. Some games are relaxing, but others stimulate the brain if it is a logic-based game, whereas games where the character is constantly running around will build up your stress due to the pace and adrenaline involved.

Stress is a major form of indigestion. Many people who suffer from lack of sleep would say that it is due to the daily worries of work or their families, for example. A common problem today is being unable to switch off. Anxiety, worry, depression, unpleasant memories, and fears are the most common cause of sleeplessness. They seem to take on a life of their own when you are left in silence and they are determined to keep you awake, even though it is often the middle of the night.

The third common cause of insomnia, one that has become common only in more modern times, is tampering with the normal cycle of sleeping and waking. This is a mechanical problem of sorts. Human beings have a normal sleep rhythm - in general, we are designed to be awake in daylight and asleep at night. People who work night shifts, or travellers who have recently crossed several time zones, may experience a great deal of insomnia simply because they are trying to sleep when their internal clock is telling their body to be awake.

Our bodies are designed for sleep to come effortlessly. When it doesn't, there are a number of ways of inducing the body and mind to let go and slip gently into a restful sleep.

Creating an environment to help sleep

This should be done in conjunction with the practice of yoga, but should be discussed as it is one of the main motivations for someone taking up yoga. Your bedroom should be tranquil and inviting. You should aim to make it as comfortable and encouraging to sleep in. you should try to eliminate any ambient light and any noise that has the potential to disturb your sleep. If possible, you should reserve the bedroom for sleep. Conduct other activities-reading, watching TV, paying bills, and disciplining your children-in another room. In time, this will create the expectation in your body that the bedroom is where it goes to relax and rest.

End the day calmly!

You should always aim to go to bed at about the same time every night, whether or not you are going to work the next day. You should also create some form of routine that will prepare you for a night of sleep. You may already have some kind of programme that you follow before you go to bed, which includes locking the house, brushing your teeth, reading, switching all the lights off. A pre-bed routine is a very effective way of telling your unconscious that it is time for you to go to sleep.

It is important for you to make sure that this routine is relaxing, and in no way stimulating. Winding down before bed time will help to increase the likelihood that your mind will let you rest. If you find the news on TV or radio disturbing, you should never watch the late broadcast before you go to bed. If you live in a safe area, it is highly recommended to take a leisurely walk to tire you out to an extent. You could also try to read something pleasant and soothing. In other words, you should save the suspense novel for reading earlier in the day. Take a hot bath and, more importantly, try to sit for a period of meditation. The trick is to try to calm your mind and quieten down your nerves before you even get as far as climbing into bed.

Finally, getting up at the same time every morning will make it far easier to fall asleep at night. If you try to compensate for a night of disturbed sleep by staying in bed longer in the morning, you will simply disrupt your sleep cycle even further. You should always get up on time, even if you don't feel like you've had enough rest, because you will have a much better chance of falling asleep easily when bedtime comes around again.

Doing relaxation exercises

Taking a few minutes to do a short relaxation exercise just before getting into bed is an excellent way of letting go. This doesn't have to be elaborate. Great benefits can be gained by simply lying on your back in the corpse pose (with your hands at your sides, palms facing upwards, and feet slightly apart). Close your eyes, and systematically address every part of your body. Start at your scalp and move toward your toes. Begin by softening your forehead, eyes, face, and jaw. Tensing and then releasing each muscle group help tight muscles to loosen off, especially those in the neck and shoulders. Continue giving attention to each area of your body-the arms, the trunk, and the legs-until you reach your toes. Try to surrender to the gravity surrounding you.

Stay in this relaxed state for a few minutes, letting the floor support you. Focus on your breathing, releasing all other concerns. Let your breath come from deep in your abdomen, and let it flow smoothly, slowly, and evenly. This simple exercise is a way of telling your mind and body that it is OK to stop thinking, working, and struggling.

Pay close attention to what you eat

It is always best to eat a light meal in the evening, especially if you are dining late. You will sleep far more deeply if you have completely finished digesting your food before you go to bed. A rich, heavy meal close to bedtime will interfere with your rest and leave you feeling very sluggish in the morning.

You should try to avoid caffeine, especially after midday. This includes coffee, tea, chocolate, and many sodas. Coffee has a half-life of four to six hours, which means that it takes that long for half of the coffee to be digested, and another four to six hours for the next quarter of it to be eliminated from your body. In other words, it takes twelve to fourteen hours for most of the coffee you have drunk to be eliminated. That is why you may often still feel wide awake at bed time when you had your last cup of tea or coffee after dinner.

Sugar can also cause problems with sleep. It is always beneficial to consider avoiding refined sugar in the evening because it is absorbed immediately into the bloodstream. That's why it gives you a burst of energy and sometimes makes you feel a little high. Eating sugar near bedtime can make you restless and jittery and can keep you from falling asleep. If you need a treat at bedtime, a glass of warm milk is your best bet.

Alcohol and tobacco taken near bedtime can also interfere with deep sleep. It is true that a night cap will make you sleepy, but the sleep it induces is light, restless, and shot through with periods of wakefulness. Likewise, you may associate tobacco with relaxation, but it actually increases tension. Tobacco is a stimulant that makes the heart race and blood pressure rise. It's best avoided altogether, but if you choose to smoke, avoiding it in the hour or two before bedtime will make your sleep more restful.

Take some exercise

it is a fact that people who undertake manual work for most of the day, such as builders or farmers, have far fewer problems with insomnia. Sufferers are more commonly housewives, office workers and anyone else who does a stressful job, such as medical staff. For most of us, hard work is reserved for the brain, so it is essential for us to exercise our bodies if we're going to have the possibility of sleeping well. Studies of athletes have shown that they do not require more (or less) sleep than less-exercised people, but their ratio of deep to light sleep is far higher. In other words, they need the same amount of sleep as the rest of us, but their sleep is far less disturbed, and much more satisfying. Doing some form of aerobic exercise at least three times a week will help you to increase this ratio. Just be sure to avoid strenuous exercise within several hours of bedtime because it can have the effect of being stimulating. But if you exercise at any other time, you'll sleep better.

It is OK to do long, slow stretches near bedtime, however, for they will serve to release muscular tension and prepare you for sleep. Focus on asanas that you find relaxing. Avoid intense backward bends, such as the wheel, as they may prove to be far too invigorating at the end of the day.

Do not take medicines to help you sleep!

According to a recent article in the American magazine, Archives of Internal Medicine, approximately 20 million prescriptions are written all over the world each year for sleeping aids, such as Valium. This number is actually far less than the actual number of people taking sleeping aids, as they are readily available as over the counter medicines. Although most of these drugs do help to bring about sleep within ten to twenty minutes, they can actually interfere with the deeper stages of sleep. And all of them impair functioning the next day in one way or another. They can be helpful for short-term insomnia resulting from a sudden stressful event, but even the mainstream medical community agrees that sleep medications and sedatives are not helpful in resolving chronic sleep problems for any length of time.

Try Homeopathic remedies

Homeopathic remedies and herbs can help with
insomnia, and they do not disturb other areas of your
sleep or of your life. Homeopathic medicines are
extremely dilute extracts from natural substances, so
they don't have the rebound effects drugs do. They
are considered to be non-toxic by the FDA, and many
low-potency remedies are sold over the counter. One
of the best treatments for insomnia is homeopathic
coffee, called coffea cruda. Although coffee causes
irritability and sleeplessness in physiologic doses, in
homeopathic doses it can cure these states.

Valerian root, passionflower, and hops, taken
before bedtime in either tablet or tea form, are other
alternatives to aid your sleep. These gentle, relaxing
substances help your body rest, but they don't affect
your central nervous system the way prescription
sleep medicines do. Both homeopathic remedies and
herbal preparations can be purchased at most health
food stores or through a holistic physician.

In summary...

Insomnia is a huge problem in this fast-paced, sugar
and caffeine addicted country. But if we can first
identify the habits we have that contribute to our
sleeplessness and begin to slowly change them, and at
the same time add more relaxation and deep
breathing to our pre-sleep routine, we will ultimately
sleep better.

Above all, don't panic. Insomnia is not a life-threatening condition, although many people respond to it with agitation or fear. The more anxious you make yourself about not sleeping, the more sleep will escape you. So you should turn the clock to the wall and stop thinking about the conversation in your mind about what a horrible day you will have tomorrow if you don't get to sleep immediately. The key to sound sleep lies in surrendering, not in trying harder. Once you are in bed, focus on your breathing and empty your mind. If you have a mantra, let your mind rest in it. Be kind to yourself! Always remember, sleep cannot be forced, but it can be coaxed.

Yoga as a benefit for children

Children today are under a lot more stress than those many years ago. Homework, pressure to compete with other children, endless after-school activities, all adds up, just like it does in adults. And just like their parents, kids today are turning to Yoga to help them to relax. This is a great way for them to do so, as the exercising will not strain them unnecessarily, and will not have an adverse effect on their little growing bodies.

Yoga can help them develop far better body awareness, self-control, flexibility and co-ordination. It can also allow them to carry these skills beyond the class and into their daily routines. For example, breathing exercises can help children immensely when they are faced with homework for each of their school subjects. If they have learned how to breath properly and effectively, their stress will go within a few minutes.

Yoga has also been shown to help children who are hyperactive and have an attention deficit. These children crave movement and sensory stimulus. Yoga can help them to channel these impulses in a positive way. Yoga poses that seem to work especially well are the warrior pose and tree pose. They help instil calmness, confidence and balance. The trick with children is to get beyond simply 'doing' the posture. They need to think about what the postures mean, to become like the postures - strong and confident like a warrior. Working with others, the children also manage to develop team skills and bonding with others.

When it comes to sleeping and relaxation – just as with adults – some children have a difficult time closing their eyes while others can't get enough. One technique that encourages relaxation is visualisation. First, they might focus on stomach breathing and listening to relaxing music. Then they might continue their yogic development by imagining that they are at the beach, or playing their favourite sport, or doing some other activity that they like. At the end of the relaxation exercise, they should be encouraged to share their own experiences and discuss why they helped.

Asanas for helping with PMS or PMT

Almost every woman experiences symptoms of pre menstrual syndrome (PMS), otherwise known as pre-menstrual tension (PMT) at one time or another. Precisely why is still an open question in the medical field, although both Ayurvedic and homeopathic physicians have suggested that lifestyle factors that disrupt the body's natural rhythm and create hormonal imbalances will play a significant role, as well as the simple hormonal changes with the onset of menstruation (or a period). Stress, bad eating habits, travelling, overwork, difficulties in relationships, and lack of exercise all contribute to the pattern of emotional instability, anxiety, irritability, depression, and mood swings, which is characteristic of PMS. These symptoms are often accompanied by headaches, food cravings, weight gain, bloating, breast tenderness, and a host of other unpleasant physical symptoms.

PMS has been classified and grouped into four different types – Type A (anxiety), Type C (craving), Type D (depression), and Type H (H_2O retention). The anxiety that characterises Type A is the one that is often accompanied by irritability and mood swings. In addition to experiencing cravings-notably for sugar (mainly chocolate) – those who have Type C PMS often have fatigue and headaches. Confusion and even memory loss frequently accompany the depression that is the distinguishing feature of Type D. The water retention characteristic of Type H PMS can also cause weight gain, bloating, and breast tenderness. This is not to say that a woman will experience only one type of PMS or that her symptoms will be the same each month. Any combination of these symptoms may occur. They will vary from month to month depending on which stress is present and which hormone predominates.

Doctors in LA have developed a complete treatment model based on the four main types of PMS as outlined above. The self-help measures that they recommend include moderate exercise, dietary changes and supplements, massage, and yoga postures. Because yoga postures provide both immediate relief for the discomfort of PMS and an opportunity for inner renewal, they will be the focus here. The postures suggested are based on those which will specifically help PMS, but it is obviously useful to practice them alongside other postures, not on their own.

Type A Asanas

The corpse pose (shavasana), the crocodile (makarasana), and the child's pose (balasana) are particularly helpful in relieving anxiety and nervous irritability. All three, as previously explained, are simple relaxation postures. The crocodile is helpful for women who experience severe cramping or are unable to relax lying on their backs. It allows the mind to focus inward with fewer distractions as the head faces downward, like a crocodile concealed underwater. The child's pose is a compact foetal like posture that relaxes the body completely. It focuses the breath on the organ systems in the abdomen and pelvis, which helps massage and tone them. The gentle inversion of head, neck, and torso relaxes the back muscles, therefore easing low back pain, which is a common pre menstrual complaint.

Doing a systematic deep relaxation exercise in either the corpse or crocodile pose calms and soothes the nervous system. This relaxation exercise can be self-directed or done while listening to a tape. When doing a relaxation exercise, you must always remember to close the eyes and keep your focus inward. Let go of any mental clutter and be aware of the breath and how it is moving in and out of your body. Always make sure that you are breathing from your diaphragm and that the breath flows smoothly and evenly through the nostrils without noise or jerks.

The Corpse Pose to do this, you should begin by lying on your back, your arms at your sides, palms up, and your feet a comfortable distance apart. Always be sure to adjust your head, neck, and shoulders to bring them into alignment with the rest of your body. Close your eyes and relax and allow the floor to support you. Always remember to breathe deeply and from the diaphragm.

The Crocodile Lie on your abdomen with your head tucked inward and down and your forehead resting on top of your folded fore arms. The legs should be a comfortable distance apart, with your feet and toes pointing outward. Always breathe fully, feeling the abdomen expanding downward with each inhalation and your hips and buttocks rising slightly upward with the exhalation. Allow the gentle movement to soothe your pre menstrual cramping and massage the uterine muscles.

The Child's Pose As previously, you should kneel with your buttocks resting on your heels. Bend at the hips and let your torso relax on your thighs and your forehead rest on the floor. Relax your arms and hands on the floor beside you with the palms up and the fingers pointing toward your feet. Place a pillow either on your lap if you are having difficulty folding your body over your thighs, or between your calves and thighs if you cannot rest comfortably on your heels.

Type C Asanas

Many women experience food cravings before the onset of menstruation, especially cravings for sugar and chocolate. The body needs much more glucose that usual because it is more responsive to insulin at this time and may translate this need into a craving for sweets. Chocolate contains magnesium, a mineral that decreases menstrual cramping and helps to regulate glucose metabolism. The problem with using sugar and chocolate to meet these nutritional needs is that consuming them often induces a let-down feeling, fatigue, and headaches-all of which are characteristic of Type C PMS.

Two postures that stimulate blood flow to the abdominal and pelvic areas and help regulate sugar metabolism are the bow (dhanurasana) and the modified bridge (setu bandha). The bow stretches and tones the ovaries, uterus, and abdominal organs. The upward momentum created by the sweeping movement of the head, eyes gazing toward the sky, and legs drawn up, increases energy and elevates the mood. Performing the modified bridge with controlled breathing rejuvenates and tones the reproductive organs as well as the abdominal organs, thereby helping to relieve carbohydrate cravings.

The Bow Lying face down with your arms at your sides, bend your legs at the knees and bring your feet toward your buttocks. Clasp your ankles and raise your trunk off the floor. Squeeze your buttocks together and bring your knees in close to each other. Hold the pose 10 to 15 seconds and repeat up to 3 times.

The Modified Bridge Lie on your back with your knees bent, your feet parallel to each other and close to your buttocks. Rest your arms at your sides with your palms down. On the exhalation, elongate your spine by pressing your lower back into the floor. Inhaling, lift your pelvis and then your mid-back and upper back. Your weight is now supported by your shoulders and feet. Hold the pose for 10 to 15 seconds. Roll down by slowly lowering the upper back to the floor, followed by the mid-back and pelvis. Repeat this gentle flexing of the spine, rolling up and down 5 or 6 times.

Type D Asanas

Because the bow has a mood-elevating and rejuvenating effect, it is also excellent for women suffering from Type D PMS as well for those with Type C symptoms. The upward-facing dog (urdhva mukha shvanasana), which is also a backward-bending pose, stimulates both the back and front of the body, especially the lumbar and pelvic regions. The upward gaze and sweeping movement towards the sky not only counteracts the downward pull of gravity, but also helps relieve depression.

The Upward-facing Dog   Begin in a prone position, forehead on the floor, arms bent at the elbows next to your chest, fingers pointing forward, elbows in. On an inhalation, begin rising up from the forehead, nose, and chin, continuing the stretch through your neck, upper torso, and lower torso until your entire pelvic basin is tilting upward. Feel the weight shift as you start supporting yourself on your arms. Gradually straighten the arms, broadening your shoulders down and away from the ears, stretching and curving your spine, and tightening your buttocks. Your weight is supported on the tops of your feet and your hands. Keep the backside firm and lifting up. Hold for 30 seconds to 1 minute.

Type H Asanas

Gentle inversion postures have been found to be most helpful for problems of weight gain, bloating, and tender breasts. The modified wide-angle pose (upavishtha konasana) and the half or supported plough (halasana) are two gentle, effective postures for relieving the symptoms of Type H PMS.

The modified wide-angle pose relieves swelling by opening and energising the entire pelvic region. By directly altering the pull of gravity, it reverses the effects of bloating and fluid retention in the legs and feet. The half or supported plough pose similarly reduces swelling and fluid retention by stimulating circulation in an inverted position. The modified version of the posture is recommended over the full plough here to avoid injury to the lower back-the muscles in the lumbar area are already stressed due to the pressure caused by fluid build-up in the pelvic basin.

The wide angle pose   Lie on your back with your pelvis against a wall, your legs extended up the wall, and your arms resting at your sides. Open your legs into a V on the wall. Breathe easily, holding this position for 1 minute. Then bring your legs together and hold them straight up for another minute. Repeat the cycle twice more.

The Half Plough From a supine position, raise your legs over your head until they are parallel to the floor. Support your hips and back with your hands, arms bent, elbows tucked next to your rib cage. Hold the pose for up to 3 minutes, depending on how comfortable you are. Come out of the pose by bending your knees close to your forehead and rolling down, making contact with the floor one vertebra at a time.

You may wish to rest your feet on a prop such as a chair or a stack of pillows to relieve any strain in the lumbar region.

Many of us sail through our monthly cycles barely noticing changes in our physical and mental states. But those of us whose bodies are uncomfortable and agitated with each hormonal shift are given a special opportunity to renew ourselves each month. This is the perfect time to turn to yoga practice.

Pain release through yoga

Yoga is more commonly being used as an aid to
easing pain and chronic pain. This could be an injury
caused by a road traffic accident, or could be pain
associated with an illness, such as arthritis. Other
conditions which can benefit many times over
through the practice of yoga are those connected with
the spine. This is because most of yoga centres
around the bending and stretching of the spine in a
gentle and moderate way. The art will also allow you
to become at peace internally – which is the key to
being at peace externally. Patanjali in his classic
scripture the Yoga Sutras describes this as a balance of
steadiness, or sthira, and comfort, or sukha.

During the first few sessions, it is important to try
to access sthira and sukha through the release of
some of the tension in the foundations of your body.
You should learn to find, feel, and relax your pelvic
floor, buttocks, stomach , anal, and genital areas. You
must next learn to isolate and lift the centre of your
pelvic floor – the perineum – while relaxing the
surrounding muscles. With coaching you will be able
to continue the lift through the centre of your body,
connecting the perineal lift to a subtle lift in his
abdomen, sternum, and the crown of your head. This
'core lift' will begin to give you an internal strength
that your body can begin to relax into.

To further enhance the benefits, this practice of

core lift should always be co-ordinated with dirgha
and ujjayi pranayama, which are, three-part sounding
breaths. Finally, you must practice how to breathe
into the pain, experience it as a sensation. It is also a
good time to point out that if you are suffering from
any form of pain, you will have an emotional barrier
built up to protect yourself from allowing it to take
over your life completely. You should therefore use
yoga to allow yourself to release some of the
emotional armour that has added stress to you mind
and your body. This practice can be enhanced by
learning to 'talk' and 'listen' to your body once and
for all. This will help you to discover any underlying
negative attitudes, which you will then be able to
transform into proper and sympathetic ways of
healing.

You should practice this at home, and you will
find that you are able to go deeper into the pain
without tensing up, and you will become familiar
enough with your body to find and sustain the core
lift without any assistance. You will find very quickly
that you will experience an increase in awareness,
confidence, and muscle tone in the core of your body.

When you are injured, the muscles and tissue that
protect the moving parts of your body-the joints-try
to stabilise you by tightening in spasm. Most
treatments focus on releasing the spasm, but if there's
no core strength to rest on, the spasm may return. As
you learn to develop core strength through the

practice of yoga, parts of your body that were chronically contracted will finally begin to relax into an internal support. For the first time you was able to breathe into your pain and release some of the emotional protection you are carrying.

It is clear that Yoga can effectively release chronic pain. But you must have a willingness to be in a new relationship with your body and its pain, have a compassionate and supportive intention, and develop core strength. The following exercise may be of benefit to you...

Preparing the body with conscious breathing

The first step is to establish full, deep breathing. Use the sounding breath and the three-part breath pranayama in combination with each other.

When you have chronic pain, breathing tends to be shallow and you frequently hold your breath. With this restricted breathing, you are not exhaling fully and therefore cannot remove from the lungs stale air and the residual build up of toxins. With chronic pain, the muscles are cold and contracted from poor circulation, so even less oxygen comes in and fewer toxins are removed. In other words, it is a vicious circle – one worsens the other.

When you breathe fully and deeply, the lungs work more, the diaphragm moves and the inter costal, back, and abdominal muscles work. This generates heat into the core of the body.

Another positive result of conscious breathing is its calming effect on the emotions, reducing fear and anxiety in the nervous system. You feel safer emotionally as well as more at ease and relaxed physically. Conscious breathing also helps diminish tension before it accumulates around the areas where chronic pain exists.

Establish a supportive mental attitude

The next step in releasing chronic pain involves changing your attitude towards the part of the body which is in pain. You should really aim to observe not only what the pain feels like, but how you actually feel about the pain. The intention is for you to feel the emotions connected with the part of the body that hurts. This important step connects emotional pain with physical pain, and enables you to recognise the continuity between your body, mind, and feelings. There are many attitudes associated with chronic pain: suffering, anger, despair, depression, loss, and helplessness, to name a few. These attitudes exist when we hate, fear, or deny parts of our body that hurt. Because we cannot simply remove the hurt, we begin to hide and shield ourselves from it, denying it the attention and love it actually needs to heal. This of course adds to the stress because of the negative self-directed energy required to deny parts of ourselves.

The first step in changing the negative attitude is

Yoga and Health Benefits

to create a feeling of comfort and safety. Begin by placing yourself into a comfortable, relaxed position, lying on the floor in the relaxation pose, or maybe in a restorative posture. Force yourself to begin to communicate with the pain by placing a hand on the part of the body that hurts.

Putting hands on the painful part of the body is soothing. It opens a relationship to this part and brings a message that you are willing to make a different choice in your relationship with it – you are not simply trying to ignore it. It will start to send energy, heat, and fluid to this part of the body, creating an overall feeling of well-being and help. It will invite the painful part of the body to rejoin the rest of the you and will help move you from the feelings of denial to interest.

The next stage is to breathe into the part of the body being touched and actually feel what is going on, and ask if it has a voice. If so, you should then ask the body to speak to you. You will very probably feel anger, despair, and will judge what is going on in a negative way. Your whole self will probably be in denial physically, mentally, and emotionally. You will more than likely feel as if your body has betrayed you and you will feel angry with it for doing so. You will also feel confused as to why this has happened to you, and may even feel like a failure for not being able to deal with it.

At this point in the process, there will often be a

release – you will begin to come out of the feelings of denial. There is a wide range of emotional releases, from full expression to silence. Now is the time to use affirmations because your critical language will keeps the pain where it is for longer. You should at this point restate how you feel after the release, for instance that you now feel as if you are getting to know the pain in that part of your body. This will help you show yourself that your feelings are changing between mind and body.

Increasing intimacy and awareness of the body

Once you have released some of the emotional protection and have begun to move beyond denial, the next step is to release chronic tension substantially by using specific Yoga movements combined with your breath.

Our culture tends to strengthen on top of unrecognised vulnerability and helplessness; we go in quickly, name the pain, and get out. But true strength runs much deeper and can only take root in the vulnerability- it is crucial that you are able to go to the centre of what is inside if you are truly going to heal properly. To do this you need to create a balance of steadiness and comfort with core stability and strength.

To build core strength a strong and mobile pelvic floor, a softly engaged abdomen, an open, lifted heart, and an aligned spine are essential. Pelvic floor work provides the foundation anatomically, neurological, structurally, and energetically.

The pelvic floor relates to the muladhara or root chakra where basic issues of survival and safety reside. If this part of the body is frozen then the foundation of safety is locked and movement is based in fear. When you begin to stretch open the pelvic floor, energy can move through and up this chakra, and you can consciously act on issues of survival and fear, thus building a strong foundation for living.

Stretching open, moving, and strengthening the pelvic floor is followed by a unique movement, called the core lift, by which the centre of the pelvic floor – the perineum – is subtly lifted up into the core of the body. In various yogic texts this is called mulabandha. Please note at this point that there are different schools of thought as to what does and does not constitute mulabandha. For our purposes, mulabandha does not include the lifting and contraction of the genitals, vajroli mudra, or the lifting and contracting of the anus, ashvini mudra. It also is not the form of mulabandha that is only practised in a meditative sitting posture, such as siddhasana, with retention of the breath, kumbhaka, and application of the throat lock, jalandhara bandha.

It is important to note that the pelvic floor is not an easy part of the body to access because our culture associates it with pain, shame, inappropriateness, and sin. And for some of us there is trauma in this area from surgery and/or sexual abuse. These issues make it more difficult to bring to this part of the body an unfettered curiosity. Most Yoga teachers are not experienced or trained to relate in depth with this type of trauma, so as a Yoga teacher has to know their limits and be capable and confident, because once this type of problem is surfaced, they must be prepared to stay with it and bring in a professional or suggest professional therapy if appropriate.

The core lift is accomplished by a subtle lifting or arching of the pelvic floor into the core of the body. This is done by contracting the muscles surrounding the perineum, the area between the genitals and the anus. It's not difficult to do, yet because the lift is subtle it requires as much attention and focus as any technique in Yoga. The ability to focus, however, is of great benefit because when our mind is strongly focused, we can begin to relax and feel safe.

Yoga for MS

Multiple Sclerosis is an auto immune disease in which the body's defensive immune system attacks and destroys the fatty tissue – or myelin – surrounding nerves in the brain and spinal cord. These myelin sheaths perform the same function as insulation around an electrical wire. Without the myelin insulation, nerve impulses from brain to body can short out and become confused, misdirected, or be completely blocked. Symptoms can include numbness and/or tingling in the extremities, weakness, lack of co-ordination and/or balance, gait difficulties, slurring of speech, blurred or double vision, bowel and bladder dysfunction, vertigo, and heat intolerance.

Physical activity is extremely important for individuals with MS, and yoga is now recognised as an excellent means of MS management, whether the individual shows little or no outward signs of the disease, or whether they spend most of their time in a wheelchair.

The benefits of yoga postures (asana), working with the breath (pranayama), and meditation may include increased body awareness, release of muscular tension (thus relieving spasticity), increased co-ordination and balance, increased flexibility and strength, control over fatigue, increased tolerance to heat, improved circulation and breathing, improved organ function (including bowel and bladder), enhanced alertness, better management of stress and an overall feeling of well-being.

The course of MS is unpredictable. The four categories used to classify the clinical course in persons with MS are: Relapsing-remitting, Primary-progressive, Secondary-progressive, Progressive-relapsing. The following is a brief description of how yoga can help with these categories of MS.

Relapsing-Remitting
In the category of Relapsing-remitting MS, after an initial flare-up and diagnosis of MS, the patient will tend to have extended periods with mild flare-ups and minor disease progression. The symptoms generally include numbness and tingling, some balance issues, and heat intolerance. In addition to yoga, patients will usually receives injections.

It is normal for a gentle practice to be developed for students with MS, to avoid overheating the body, but if you have been used to an active or vigorous lifestyle, the practice can include a modified Flow Series of standard postures linked by a sun salutation. To avoid tiring yourself, however, you must ensure that you practice this series slowly, mindfully, and with complete awareness. In this way the practice becomes more meditative and less fatiguing, but still invigorating and relaxing. You will probably have a well-developed sense of body awareness, so you will be able to let your teacher know when the practice is too much for yourself. Meditative or cooling pranayama practices such as Shitali, Nadi Sodhana, and Pratiloma Ujjayi should also be included in the practice, as well as a long guided imagery meditation at the end of each session.

Over a period of time, when the yoga is being used and developed, you will find that you will develop an increased ability to handle stressful situations and have a much more balanced perspective about your life. You may find that, fairly quickly, you will spend more and more time without a flare up occurring.

Secondary-Progressive

In the category of Secondary-progressive MS, you will experience a relapsing-remitting disease course at the outset, which will be followed by a more steady progression. The symptoms may include near-blindness, severe vertigo when reclining, slurred speech, and muscle weakness. You will more than likely be able to transfer from her wheelchair into a folding chair, so that's where most of the yoga work should be done, often using two chairs to simulate working on the floor. A modified version of seated forward bends (paschinmottanasa, janu sirsasana), seated backbends (matsyasana, yoga mudra), hip openers (badha konasana), twists (ardha matsyendrasana), and modified standing postures such as forward bends (uttanasana, padottanasana), should be used, along with a variation of warrior (virabadrasana II). This treatment should also include strong breath awareness to allow your diaphragm to begin working again and to get some life-force stirring up inside of you .

The primary objective here is to help to regain muscle strength and flexibility which has been lost to years of being in a wheelchair – this can work extremely well. You may eventually even been able to stand for brief periods of time.

Progressive-Relapsing

Progressive-relapsing MS is a problem where your range of motion is often limited to simply being able to move your head, some lifting of your shoulders, and moving of your arms and hands only very slightly. In this case, it is a good idea to have some hands-on manipulation, where appropriate, of the arms, hands, and legs. But mainly, the work should centre on mindful breathing (ujjayi, viloma and anoloma pranayama), dynamic movement of the head, shoulders and arms linked to breath, and guided imagery meditation to promote mindfulness and relaxation.

In many cases, the obvious physical limitations exclude even a modified physical yoga practice to a great degree. However, as we already know, yoga does not stop at the physical level. It spills into the other aspects of our being, such as the energetic, mental, emotional, and spiritual aspects (the koshas). Work with sufferers of this type of MS may serve to improve the quality of their life in all these levels, even though the physical practice may not look like 'yoga' to an outsider.

Never limit yourself to the physical alone. Utilise breath work, mindfulness based meditation, guided imagery, and experiment gently to find the appropriate practice for yourself, keeping in mind your needs and desires.

The use of yoga for facial exercise

Your face works very hard and is often neglected. It helps you see, breathe, chew, speak, laugh, cry, kiss, grin, grimace, smile, frown, sneeze and a lot more. It gets hit by sun, rain, wind, snow, rubs, scratches, scrapes, make-up, grit and grime, as well as smiles, stares, glares and other looks from friends, family and strangers.

Your face deserves to be treated to the positive effects of yoga too. The following are a few simple face exercise that will help to relax tense muscles, release stress and improve circulation.

- **Palming** – Find a comfortable seated position, either on floor on a cushion or in a chair. Sit with your back straight. Begin with your eyes closed. Focus on your breath as it moves in and out of your nostrils. Always remember to think of your breathing as being cool air in, warm air out. Next, rub your palms together very fast until they feel warm. Then cup them over your closed eyes. Repeat.

  The benefits of this include the soothing of the optic nerve, eyes and area around the eyes.

- **The Great Rub** -- Place the index and middle fingers of both hands in the middle of your forehead. Rub your forehead by making small circles with your fingers. Next, move your fingers across your brow and to your temples, pausing there to give them a gentle massage. This is an area where you hold stress and tension that can often lead to headaches. Next, move down from your temples to the hinge of your jaw, pausing to massage your jaw muscles. From there, move across your cheeks and up along the side of your nose to your forehead. Repeat.

The benefits of this include the release of stress and tension, particularly in the temples and jaw areas.

- **Eye socket massage** – Take your index and middle fingers of each hand and place them on either side of your nose just below the bridge. Rub your fingers up to the bridge of your nose and along your eyebrows. You'll feel a notch in your eye socket where the bone begins to turn downward. Rub the notch gently for a moment. Then follow the line of the socket rim down beneath the eye and back up along the side of your nose. Repeat 3-5 times.

The benefits of this include the relaxation of the eyes and surrounding areas, and it will also relieve stress and tension.

- **Clenched smile** – Grit your teeth and open your lips as wide as they will go. Feel your lips, cheeks,

chin and neck stretch to their limit. Hold...and
release. Repeat.

The benefits of this include the increase of
circulation, relaxation of faces muscles, relieving
stress and tension.

- **Scrunches** – Scrunch your face real tight. Purse
  your lips, draw your cheeks in toward your nose,
  pull your eye brows down and bring the flesh of
  your chin up toward your mouth. Hold...and
  release. Repeat.

  The benefits include providing a counter
  stretch to the 'Clench' exercise. It will also increase
  circulation, relax faces muscles, relieving stress
  and tension.

- **The Lion** – Take a deep breath. All at once, exhale
  forcefully, open your mouth wide, stick your
  tongue out as far as it will go, say "Aghhhhhhh,"
  and open your eyes wide and look up. Repeat 3
  times.

  This is a very effective yoga exercise to do
  because it relieves tension in the throat and face
  and stimulates the eyes and improves circulation.

- **Cheek Pinch** – Pinch your cheeks, by grabbing
  bits of flesh and giving them a squeeze to improve
  the circulation in your face.

CHAPTER 5
Moving on

Combining asanas

When you have spent some time becoming familiar
with the asanas described above, so that you can
perform them without the book, finding yourself
more and more supple each time you do them, you
will be able to plan your use of them. It is not for one
moment suggested that you attempt to do all of them
every time you practice yoga, while to follow the
same routine day in day out would not only become
tedious but restrict the value of yoga to your overall
health.

However you combine asanas in your regular
routine, it is wise to start with some simple rolling
and stretching exercises as a way of warming your
muscles. If you then went on to the Sun Salutation,
you could be sure of thoroughly warming up before
moving on to other postures.

Some people like to work all on one level in a

215

session: for instance, a session of all standing or all sitting or all lying-down postures. There is nothing wrong with this as long as you remember that within yoga every pose has a counter-pose, and the point of this is balance: if you are stretching and working muscles hard in one direction, you need then to work them in the other direction too. So, for instance, if you do the Bridge, you should balance this by doing a forward bend, or the Cat or Dog, for example. The Fish pose is usually followed by the Corpse, and because it is so calming, most sessions end with that pose.

If you have a particular medical condition, you may want to concentrate your sessions on the postures known to benefit that. For example, if you are suffering from panic attacks or anxiety, focus on the breathing exercises as well as those offering deep relaxation such as the Corpse. If you have digestive problems, focus on spinal twists and stretches, as well as the Tree and the Plough.

Your inner health

As your sense of bodily wellbeing increases, this good effect spreads like ripples in a pond to other areas of your life. In traditional yoga practice, diet, lifestyle and meditation all have an important part to play too.

Diet

In traditional Hindu and Buddhist teachings, a vegetarian diet was an important part of the practice of yoga. The reason for this is best explained by the saying we know as 'You are what you eat'. To keep the mind clear and the body light and energetic, foods were chosen for their life and energy-giving properties, and this was felt to automatically exclude dead animal flesh. Eating meat is also contrary to the reverence for all forms of life at the heart of many Eastern religions and philosophies.

It's not the purpose of this book to encourage you to give up meat, but to suggest you look closely at your daily diet, and if necessary modify it so that your health and wellbeing are optimised. Even the most carnivorous members of the medical profession now admit that we should cut down on the amount of red meat we eat, replacing it with pulses, grains and pastas.

Whatever you feel, or don't feel, about the ethics of killing animals for food, health scares in recent years have led many people to question the factory-farming industry, where animals are raised in cramped and 'unnatural' conditions, often pumped full of hormones and other drugs to make them bigger and heavier, and forced to breed more often than nature intended. Outbreaks of listeria, E. coli and salmonella, the horror of the BSE crisis and the concurrent growth in popularity of organic foods and organic methods of food production all testify to the fact that we can't take the food on our plates for granted.

The features of a healthy diet are so well known I'm not going to repeat them in detail here. Fruit, fresh vegetables and a diet high in unprocessed carbohydrates and low in fats (including those from meat) are known to be factors in reducing the incidence of heart disease. More people die in the UK every year from heart disease than they do from cancer, and it is a simple fact that a major contributory cause of heart disease is poor diet. As a nation we are, almost literally, digging our graves with our teeth.

Yoga is not a guarantee of losing weight, but when combined with a sensible diet it can help, and certainly toned and firm limbs give an appearance of slenderness and health. It's rare to see a regular practitioner of yoga who is overweight, and the reason probably is that yoga teaches us to take good care of ourselves.

Lifestyle

It's not recommended that you practice yoga if you are under the influence of drugs or alcohol.

The so-called hard drugs, nicotine and alcohol are all powerful substances known to have a negative effect on human health. They are not only harmful to the body – both cigarettes and alcohol contribute in no small way to the yearly toll of deaths from lung and other cancers as well as heart disease – but they affect the mind, too. Alcohol, for instance, is instantly stimulating, but that toxic 'high' is followed by a crashing low; people who regularly consume large amounts of alcohol usually suffer from depression accompanied by lethargy and a joyless outlook on life.

If you are a smoker, don't regard your habit as any less addictive or dangerous than any other. It is hard to give up smoking, but your doctor, your true friends, and a host of health authorities and other agencies are keen to provide you with support in doing so. Look in a local directory or ask at your GP's surgery for contact details of smoking help lines.

Addiction of any kind wrecks your health, your life and your bank balance, but nobody should kid themselves in this hectic, pressured and very hard world that the temporary crutch afforded by any kind of drug is not attractive, nor that it is at all easy to 'just say no'.

Taking up yoga does not cure addiction, but many people have found it enormously beneficial as part of their recovery programme.

First of all, the breathing and relaxation exercises help with the tension and the panic attacks that so often either lead to the desire to pick up a drink or drugs or accompany the coming-down phase. Second, the physical asanas lead to a sense of wellbeing that helps cushion the recovering addict while coming off drugs or drink.

Third, people usually turn to drugs or drink because of inner conflicts they cannot resolve. The first stage in recovery is often an acknowledgement, followed by acceptance and understanding, of these underlying problems and the need to face them. We know how noisy the world is, how noisy we make it, and in our personal lives too we find it difficult to be still and quiet, not least because in that stillness we are faced with ourselves; sometimes we don't find ourselves the easiest of company. People with drug and alcohol problems, more than others, seek for escape and distraction from the reality of themselves. The calming, meditative aspects of yoga help settle the mind and spirit into a calm place from which to start solving problems.

Meditation

The poet T S Eliot wrote:

> *At the still point,*
> *There the dance is.*

Meditation is about tranquillity, and calm. It is about
lifting the heavy burden of work and worry and
anxiety and exhaustion off our shoulders and putting
it down for a while. It is about making an exciting
journey into the interior of ourselves. It does not have
to be complicated, or frightening. At its very simplest,
it is about making some time for yourself, and you
alone.

Meditation is very much intertwined with the
study of yoga. As yoga stretches and releases the body,
endowing it with flexibility and suppleness, so
meditation does the same for the mind. The asanas of
yoga un-knot the body; meditation untangles the
mind.

You can meditate anywhere, at any time.
Practitioners of transcendental meditation will swap
stories about having meditated on trains, standing on
Tube trains or waiting in airport lounges when they
had to. What they are doing is pressing an 'off' switch
to the world for a few moments, and pressing an 'on'
switch for themselves: I am going inside myself in
calm and quiet for a few moments. I am going to

breathe well, and in that calm and purposeful breathing I shall recover my energy.

However, most would agree that such tactics are only for emergencies. If you are going to meditate, you need a warm, quiet place in which you can be absolutely alone, a door you can shut for a while, a telephone you can switch off, somewhere to sit in comfort. If you find it comfortable to sit cross-legged on the floor, do so. You may need a cushion under your bottom, and something to rest your back against. If you prefer to sit upright on a chair, do so. You should not be slouched or slumped in a chair that is too comfy, or on a bed or sofa.

Many people like to give their meditation a special feel by using candles to light the room. Some like to construct a small 'altar' with fresh flowers, candles, incense, and perhaps one or two objects of special significance for you. Such things are important only in that they emphasise that this moment, this space, is about you – and so, of course, it is important.

Don't wear a watch. If you need to time your meditation, have a clock in the room you can check when you open your eyes – but don't have one with a loud tick. When you are absolutely silent with your eyes closed even the movement of a clock's hands can be a distraction.

Make sure you don't get cold. Wrap a blanket around your shoulders if you need to. Make sure you are not disturbed – if you live with other people, ask them to leave you alone for 15 minutes, even if there is a phone call for you (and if you can unplug the phone, do).

When you are ready, sit down, breathe well, and close your eyes. That's all it takes.

Affirmations

The purpose of mantras – a word or phrase or syllable – in meditation has been described above. They are used to focus the mind, to instil calm and to assist with the 'winding down' of meditation. It's as if the mantra spirals inwards, into the soul, and the mind follows.

Others like to begin and end their meditation with affirmations: positive sayings that encourage you and strengthen you. Examples of affirmations might be:

I am well and strong, and have faith in my life.

I am surrounded by love and peace.

I am letting go of the anger and tension in my life.

Affirmations generally begin with the words 'I am' to emphasise how the person doing the affirming is taking personal responsibility for his or her own life. Affirmations do not acknowledge chaos, disorder and disharmony; instead they say: I know I can order my own thoughts and feelings in a positive way.

Visualisation

Another tool that can be used in meditation practice is that of visualisation. As its name implies, you simply see yourself in a different place, imagine yourself there, in that circumstance, and allow that place, that sensation, to warm you and heal you.

For example, close your eyes and think of a place you particularly love. It can be a real place – somewhere you went on holiday, perhaps – or a place from your childhood, or it can be entirely imaginary, perhaps a place you have read about in a book or a poem. In your imagination, allow yourself to be there: feel your feet walking on the grass or the sand or the floor, whatever it is; feel the wind on your face; imagine every window, every blade of grass, every tree and flower.

Other people close their eyes and visualise a particular sensation that gives them pleasure. For example:

I am walking in a shower of summer rain, in the country. The rain is warm against my face and my eyelids. It's raining gently on my head, my hair, the back of my neck, my shoulders. I'm feeling clean and refreshed. If I open my lips I can taste the rain, like sweet water.

I am lying on the sand on a beach in the sun. I am the only one here. I can hear the waves coming in, washing over my feet, then pulling back into the ocean with a sigh. My shoulders and back and legs are all resting on the warm, clean sand; the sun is hot on my face, not too hot, there is a cool breeze from the sea, but I am surrounded by warmth.

There are numerous books and tapes available to help you with such exercises. On the Internet, you can look up **www.digiserve.com/gaia**. Otherwise, look in any New Age bookshop or even the larger general bookshop chains such as Borders. Health shops, even if they don't carry stock, will usually also be able to advise you.

Good luck with your yoga practice. It is good to embark on a journey that does not have an end point – yoga is for all ages and all kinds of people, it isn't something you will have to give up one day. Think of your journey as you having linked hands with millions of people down the centuries and all over the world who have, like you, taken this path to find more supple and energetic bodies and, through them, inner peace.

After the kingfisher's wing
Has answered light to light, and is silent, the light is still
At the still point of the turning world.

(T. S. Eliot)

The British Wheel of Yoga
15 Tollesby Road
Acklam
Middlesbrough
Cleveland
TS5 7PH

Yoga Therapy Centre
Royal London Homeopathic Hospial
60 Great Ormond Street
London
WC1N 3HR

Scottish Yoga Teachers Association
Frances Corr
26 Buckingham Terrace
Edinburgh
EH4 3AE

Active Birth Centre
25 Bickerton Road
London
N19 5JT
(Specialises in yoga for pregnant women)